The Management of Obesity and Related Disorders

Edited by

Peter G Kopelman MD FRCP

Professor of Clinical Medicine

Barts and the London, Queen Mary's School

of Medicine and Dentistry,

University of London,

London

UK

MARTIN DUNITZ

© Martin Dunitz Ltd 2001
First published in the United Kingdom in 2001 by

Martin Dunitz Ltd
The Livery House
7–9 Pratt Street
London NW1 0AE
UK

Tel: +44-(0)20-7482-2202
Fax: +44-(0)20-7267-0159
E-mail: info.dunitz@tandf.co.uk
Website: http://www.dunitz.co.uk

A CIP catalogue record for this book is available from the British Library

ISBN 1-85317-914-0

Distributed in the USA by
Fulfilment Center
Taylor & Francis
7625 Empire Drive
Florence, KY 41042, USA
Toll Free Tel: 1-8000-634-7064
Email: cserve@routledge_ny.com

Distributed in Canada by
Taylor & Francis
74 Rolark Drive
Scarborough
Ontario M1R 4G2, Canada
Toll Free Tel: 1-877-226-2237
Email: tal_fran@istar.ca

Distributed in the rest of the world by
ITPS Limited
Cheriton House
North Way, Andover
Hampshire SP10 5BE, UK
Tel: +44- (0)1264 332424
Email: reception@itps.co.uk

Composition by Wearset, Boldon, Tyne and Wear
Printed and bound in Great Britain by The Cromwell Press

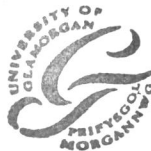

Contents

Contributors

Louise Bowles BSc MRCP
Medical Unit
Royal London Hospital
London
UK

Simon W Coppack BSc MD FRCP
Reader in Metabolic Medicine
St Bartholomew's & The Royal London School of Medicine
and Dentistry
London
UK

Jean-Pierre Després PhD
Chair Professor of Human Nutrition
Director of Research
Québec Heart Institute
Laval Hospital Research Center and
Lipid Research Center
CHUL Research Center (CHUQ)
Québec
Canada

John P Foreyt PhD
Professor, Department of Medicine
Baylor College of Medicine
Houston, TX
USA

Kenneth R Fox PhD
Professor of Exercise and Health Sciences
University of Bristol
Bristol
UK

Clare M Grace SRD MSc
Obesity Research Dietitian
Department of Diabetes and Metabolic
Medicine
St Bartholomew's & the London NHS Trust
London
UK

Ronald R Grunstein MBBS FRACP PhD MD
Clinical Associate Professor
Centre for Respiratory Failure and Sleep
Disorders
Royal Prince Alfred Hospital
Sydney
Australia

Peter G Kopelman MD FRCP
Professor of Clinical Medicine
Bart and the London, Queen Mary's School
of Medicine and Dentistry
University of London
London
UK

John G Kral MD PhD
Professor of Surgery and Medicine
Department of Surgery
SUNY Downstate Medical Center
New York, NY
USA

Isabelle Lemieux MSc
Québec Heart Institute
Laval Hospital Research Center and
Lipid Research Center
CHUL Research Center (CHUQ)
Québec
Canada

Angie Page PhD
Lecturer in Exercise and Health Sciences
University of Bristol
Bristol
UK

Antonia A Paschali MPhil
Psychology Department
University of Athens
Athens
Greece

Tracey D Robinson MBBS FRACP
Research Fellow and Associate Physician
Department of Respiratory Medicine
Royal Prince Alfred Hospital and
University of Sydney
Sydney
Australia

André J Scheen MD PhD
Professor of Medicine
University of Liège
Head of the Division of Diabetes, Nutrition
and Metabolic Disorders and Head of the
Division of Internal Medicine
Department of Medicine
CHU Sart Tilman
Liège
Belgium

John Wilding DM FRCP
Senior Lecturer in Medicine
Department of Medicine
Clinical Sciences Centre
University Hospital Aintree
Liverpool
UK

Preface

Overweight and obesity are now major problems within the developed and developing world. The associations between increasing body weight and important co-morbidities, such as cardiovascular disease, type 2 diabetes and respiratory disorders, are well recognized but effective programmes for the identification and treatment of those at particular risk are lacking. The failure of such programmes is partly explained by poor knowledge and skills of health care professionals involved in the management of overweight and obese patients.

This concise handbook presents a practical approach to the management of overweight and obese patients. It details the association between excessive fatness and medical complications and describes practical methods for successful intervention. The handbook focuses on approaches applicable in both primary and secondary care, and emphasizes the importance of a lifestyle change that includes dietary and behavioural change combined with increases in physical activity. In addition, the handbook addresses the important issues of drug treatment for obesity and surgical intervention, and provides guidance for the selection and monitoring of suitable patients. The book is intended as a practical manual for physicians in training, general practitioners and other health care professionals interested in the successful management of a serious medical condition afflicting a global population in the 21st century.

Peter G Kopelman
London, UK, 2001

Defining overweight and obesity

Peter G Kopelman

1

Introduction

Obesity is now so common within the world's population that it is beginning to replace undernutrition and infectious diseases as the most significant contributor to ill health. Major advances in the understanding of overweight and obesity have confirmed that they constitute an important medical condition. A better understanding of the genetic contribution to both weight gain and the intra-abdominal distribution of fat (central obesity) is identifying certain ethnic groups and susceptible families who are specifically at risk. In addition, there is increasing awareness that overweight and obesity are key factors in the development of other chronic diseases, in particular type 2 diabetes and coronary heart disease, and contribute to the high mortality rates of such diseases.[1] Obesity can no longer be regarded simply as a cosmetic problem affecting certain individuals, but an epidemic that requires effective measures for its prevention and management.

Definition of overweight and obesity

In clinical practice, body fat is most commonly and simply estimated by using a formula that combines weight and height. The underlying assumption is that most variation in weight for persons of the same height is due to fat mass. The formula most frequently used in epidemiological studies is body mass index (BMI) which is weight in kilograms divided by the square of the height in metres. BMI is strongly correlated with densitometry measurements of fat mass adjusted for height in middle-aged adults. The main limitation of BMI is that it does not distinguish fat mass from lean mass. The succeeding chapters on the health risks of overweight and obesity confirm that measurements of body circumference are important because excess visceral (intra-abdominal) fat is a potential risk for chronic diseases independent of total adiposity. Waist circumference and the ratio of waist circumference to hip circumference are practical measures for assessing upper body fat distribution, although neither provides a precise estimate of visceral fat. Measurement of skinfold thickness with callipers provides a more precise assessment of body fat, especially if taken at multiple sites. Skinfolds are useful in the estimation of fatness in children for whom standards have been published. However, the measurements are more difficult to make in adults (particularly in the very obese), are subject to considerable variation between observers, require accurate calipers and do not provide any information on abdominal and intramuscular fat. In general, they are not superior to simpler measures of height and weight.

Measurement of bioimpedance is based on the principle that lean mass conducts current better than fat mass because it is primarily an electrolyte solution. A measurement of the resistance to a weak current (impedance) applied across the extremities provides an estimate of body fat when combined with height and weight and an empirically derived equation. Although the devices are simple and practical to use, they neither measure fat nor predict biological outcomes more accurately than the simpler anthropometric measurements. Table 1.1 lists methods that may be used to characterize obesity.

Defining a 'healthy weight' for a particular society presents problems. There are methodological problems that derive from a definition based on total mortality rates. People frequently lose weight as a consequence of illness, unrecognized at the time of survey, that is ultimately fatal. This gives an appearance of a higher mortality among those with lower weights: reverse causation. The effect can be minimized by either excluding persons with diagnoses that might effect weight and/or those who report recent weight loss, or excluding those who die

Table 1.1
Practical clinical methods for assessment of an obese subject.

Characteristic of obesity measured	Methods
Body composition	BMI Underwater weighing Dual energy X-ray absorptiometry (DEXA) Isotope dilution Bioelectrical impedance Skinfold thickness
Regional distribution of fat	Waist circumference; waist to hip ratio Computerized axial tomography Ultrasound Magnetic resonance imaging (MRI)
Energy intake	Dietary recall or record 'Macronutrient composition' by prospective dietary record or dietary questionnaire
Energy expenditure	Doubly labelled water Indirect calorimetry (resting) Physical activity level (PAL) by questionnaire Motion detector Heart rate monitor

during the first years of follow-up. A second major concern is the confounding factors that may distort the association between body weight and mortality: cigarette smoking is of particular importance. The Nurses Health Study, which prospectively studied 116 000 women in the United States during a 17-year period, reveal a U-shaped relationship between mortality and BMI in an overall age-adjusted analysis. However, the relationship becomes a simple positive association when reverse causation is accounted for and the analysis limited to those who had never smoked.[2]

There is a close relationship between BMI and the incidence of several chronic conditions caused by excess fat: type 2 diabetes, hypertension, coronary heart disease and cholelithiasis. This relationship is approximately linear for a range of BMI indexes less than 30: American women with a BMI of 26 have a 2-fold risk of coronary heart disease compared to women with a BMI of less than 21 and an 8-fold increased risk of developing type 2 diabetes. The equivalent figures for American men are 1.5-fold increase and 4-fold increase. The risk of hypertension is doubled in both men and women with a BMI of 26. All risks are greatly increased for those subjects with a BMI >29, independent of gender.[3]

BMI can be used to estimate the prevalence of obesity within a population and the risks associated with it. It does not, however, account for the wide variation in the nature of obesity between different individuals and populations. A WHO Expert Committee has proposed the classification of overweight and obesity that applies to both men and women and to all adult age groups (Table 1.2).[4]

Waist circumference correlates with measures of risk for coronary heart disease such as hypertension or blood lipid levels. The choice of cut-off points on the waist circumference continuum involves a trade-off

between sensitivity and specificity similar to that for BMI. An expert panel has suggested increased risks if the waist circumference is >102 cm for men and >89 cm in women.[5] However, smaller cut-off points are associated with a 2- to 3-fold increase in the relative risk of type 2 diabetes. Gender-specific cut-off points for waist circumference may be of guidance in interpreting values for adults: proposed cut-off levels are shown in Table 1.3, with level 1 being intended to alert clinicians to potential risk while level 2 should initiate therapeutic action.[6] It is of critical importance to appreciate that these tables reflect knowledge acquired largely from epidemiological studies in developed countries. Preliminary information from developing nations indicates that lower cut-off levels for both BMI and waist circumference are necessary for certain populations who are at particular risk from comparatively modest degrees of overweight.

Table 1.2
Cut-off points proposed by a WHO Expert Committee for the classification of overweight. Body mass index (BMI) is the weight in kilograms divided by the height in metres.[2]

BMI (kg/m²)	WHO classification	Popular description
<18.5	Underweight	Thin
18.5–24.9	—	'Healthy', 'normal', 'acceptable'
25.0–29.9	Grade 1 overweight	Overweight
30.0–39.9	Grade 2 overweight	Obesity
≥40.0	Grade 3 overweight	Morbid obesity

Table 1.3
Gender-specific waist circumferences that denote 'increased risk' (level 1) and 'substantially increased risk' (level 2) of metabolic complications associated with obesity in Caucasians. Level 1 is intended to alert clinicians to potential risk for coronary heart disease, while level 2 should initiate therapeutic action.

	Level 1	Level 2
Men	≥94 cm	≥102 cm
Women	≥80 cm	≥88 cm

Pathophysiology of obesity

Obesity causes or exacerbates a large number of health problems, both independently and in association with other diseases. In particular, it is associated with the development of diabetes mellitus, coronary heart disease, an increased incidence of certain forms of cancer, obstructive sleep apnoea and osteoarthritis of large and small joints. The Build and Blood Pressure Study has shown that the adverse effects of excess weight tend to be delayed, sometimes for 10 years or longer.[7] Life insurance data and epidemiological studies confirm that increasing degrees of overweight and obesity are important predictors of decreased longevity.

Obesity is associated with many systemic complications (Table 1.4). Gallbladder disease is the most common form of digestive disease in obese individuals, with a progressive and linear risk from a BMI of 20 upwards. Liver abnormalities are described in obesity mainly due to fatty infiltration but, on occasion, associated with fibrosis and/or cirrhosis. Certain forms of cancer are more common in obese subjects: colorectal and prostate in obese men, carcinoma of the gallbladder, breast and endometrium in obese women. Osteoarthritis frequently accompanies obesity while bone density tends to be increased in obese subjects. Obesity in women is also associated with menstrual irregularity and infertility; obesity may be, but not always, associated with the polycystic ovary syndrome.

The succeeding chapters in this handbook address the association of increasing body weight with type 2 diabetes, dyslipidaemia, cardiovascular disease and hypertension, abnormalities of haemostasis and respiratory complications including obstructive sleep apnoea.

Table 1.4
Systemic comorbidities associated with obesity.

Cardiovascular	Hypertension
	Coronary heart disease
	Cerebrovascular disease
	Varicose veins
	Deep vein thrombosis
Respiratory	Breathlessness
	Sleep-related hypoventilation
	Sleep apnoea
	Obesity hypoventilation syndrome
Gastrointestinal	Hiatus hernia
	Gallstones
	Fatty liver and cirrhosis
	Colorectal cancer
Metabolic	Dyslipidaemia
	Insulin resistance
	Type 2 diabetes mellitus
	Hyperuricaemia
Endocrine	Increased adrenocortical activity
	Altered circulating sex steroids and binding globulin
	Breast cancer
	Polycystic ovary syndrome
	Hirsutism
Locomotor	Osteoarthritis
	Nerve entrapment
Renal	Proteinuria
Genitourinary	Endometrial cancer
	Prostate cancer
	Stress incontinence
Skin	Acanthosis nigricans
	Lymphoedema
	Sweat rashes

References

1 Kopelman PG, Obesity as a medical problem, *Nature* (2000) **404**:635–43.

2 Manson JE, Willett WC, Stampfer MJ et al, Body weight and mortality among women. *N Engl J Med* (1995) **333**:677–85.

3 Willett WC, Dietz WH, Colditz GA, Guidelines for healthy weight, *N Engl J Med* (1999) **341**:427–33.

4 World Health Organisation, *Obesity: Preventing and Managing the Global Epidemic* (WHO: Geneva, 1997).

5 World Health Organisation Expert Committee, *Physical Status: The Use and Interpretation of Anthropometry*, WHO Technical Report Series No 854 (WHO: Geneva, 1995).

6 Han TS, van Leer EM, Seidell JC, Lean MJ, Waist circumference action levels in the identification of cardiovascular risk factors: prevalence study in a random sample, *Br Med J* (1995) **311**:1401–5.

7 Lew EA, Mortality and weight: insured lives and the American Cancer Study, *Ann Intern Med* (1985) **103**:1024–9.

The Complications of Obesity

1

Obesity and diabetes

André J Scheen

2

Introduction

Besides genetic predisposition, obesity is considered as the most important risk factor for type 2 diabetes.[1,2] The strong relationship between the risk of type 2 diabetes, on the one hand, and body mass index (BMI) or weight gain, on the other hand, has been demonstrated in several studies including both men and women.[3,4] Besides the degree of obesity per se, several other factors obviously play a crucial role such as the abdominal distribution of adiposity[5,6] and the duration of overweight.[7,8] Conversely, numerous studies have demonstrated that, among obese subjects, successful weight loss results in a reduction in both the incidence and the severity of type 2 diabetes, whatever the therapeutic mean used (review in references 9 and 10).

Everybody agrees upon the fact that lifestyle modification is the cornerstone of the treatment of obese subjects with type 2 diabetes.[10] Initial recommendations to any obese diabetic patient should thus include optimization of the meal plan and enhancement of physical activity. In case of failure of conservative treatment, which unfortunately is very common, pharmacological approaches should be considered, targeting weight excess (anti-obesity agents), hyperglycaemia (anti-diabetic drugs) or both.[10–12] Attention should also be paid to the appropriate management of other risk factors frequently associated with obesity and type 2 diabetes, such as arterial hypertension and dyslipidaemias, in order to improve the poor cardiovascular prognosis of such patients.[13] Finally, when all medical approaches have failed, anti-obesity surgery may be considered in severely obese well selected diabetic patients (Figure 2.1).[9]

Etiopathogenesis of type 2 diabetes in obese subjects

It is obvious that insulin resistance plays a key role in the intimate relationship between obesity and diabetes.[14] However, not all obese subjects will develop diabetes and it is well

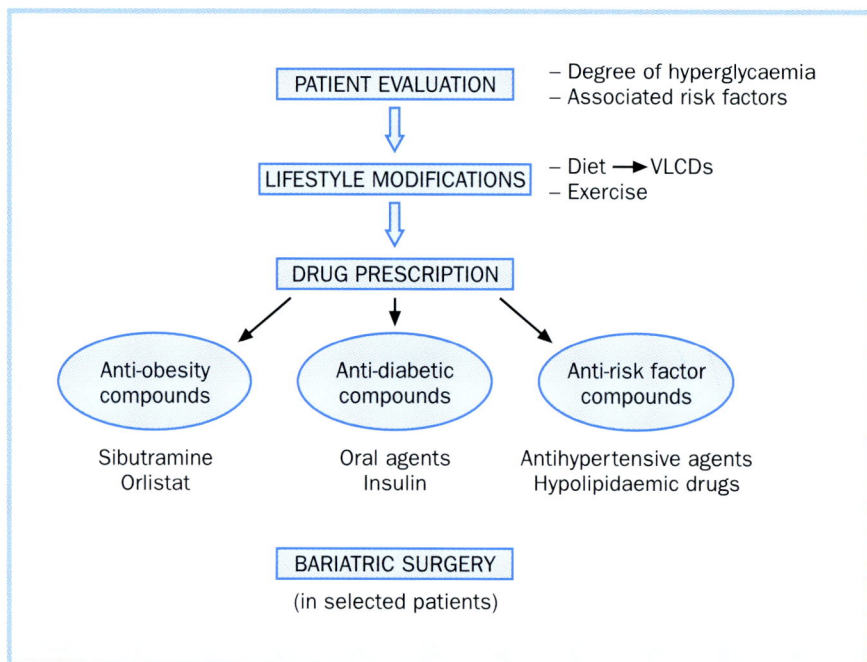

Figure 2.1
Overall management of the obese diabetic patient targeting weight excess, hyperglycaemia and other vascular risk factors. VLCDs: very-low-calorie diets (adapted from reference 10).

established that a defect in insulin secretion is mandatory for the expression of the disease.[15] Both genetic and environmental factors may be responsible for decreased insulin sensitivity and/or insulin secretion (Figure 2.2).[1,2] As one key feature of obese subjects is elevated plasma leptin levels, in proportion to increased fat mass, the potential deleterious role of this protein on insulin action and insulin secretion has been suspected.[16,17] However, despite a huge amount of recent work, the role of leptin in the development of type 2 diabetes associated with obesity remains doubtful.[18] A recent finding attributes to a new hormone called 'resistin' a crucial role in the link between obesity and diabetes.[19]

Role of insulin resistance

The presence of insulin resistance can be evidenced during various dynamic tests such as an oral glucose tolerance test (OGTT), an intravenous glucose tolerance test (IVGTT) and a euglycaemic hyperinsulinaemic

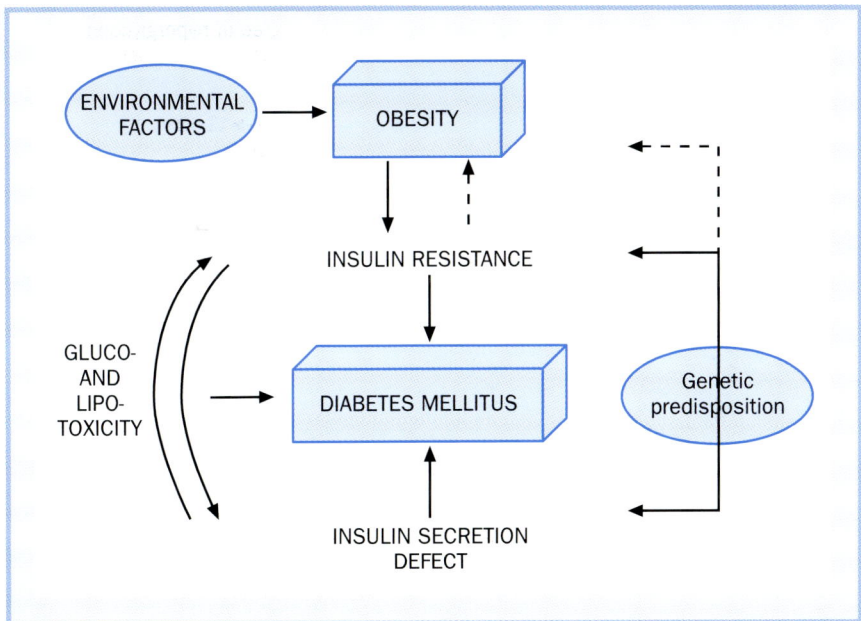

Figure 2.2
From obesity to diabetes: role of defects in insulin action and insulin secretion in the development of type 2 diabetes in genetically predisposed obese subjects (adapted from reference 15).

clamp.[20,21] The glucose clamp allows the assessment of both the insulin-mediated glucose disposal, which essentially corresponds to the utilization by the skeletal muscles, and the endogenous (hepatic) glucose production using the isotope dilution method. Changing the rate of insulin infusion, and so affecting the circulating steady-state plasma levels, facilitates the construction of dose–response curves by which decreased insulin sensitivity may be differentiated from decreased insulin responsiveness.[20] Obese non-diabetic subjects are characterized by a shift to the right of the curve depicting the relationship between insulin-stimulated glucose disposal and plasma insulin levels. In the presence of diabetes, the curve is moved further to the right and, in addition, maximal stimulation of glucose utilization is decreased, even in the presence of very high insulin levels (Figure 2.3).[22]

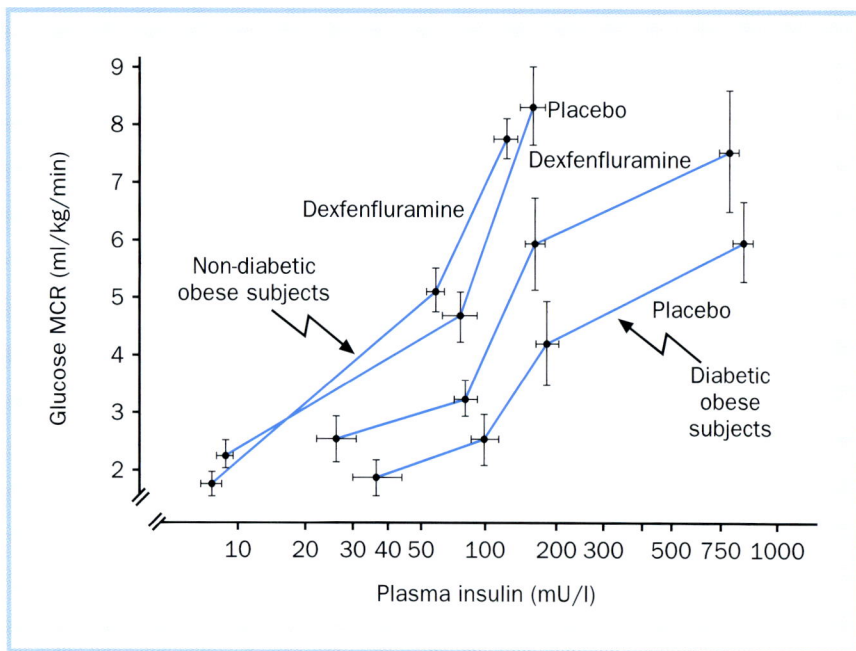

Figure 2.3
Insulin-mediated glucose disposal rates according to plasma insulin levels (logarithmic scale) in non-diabetic obese and diabetic obese subjects. Insulin resistance in obese subjects with type 2 diabetes is depicted by a right-shifted curve and a decreased maximal response. Note the significant improvement of insulin sensitivity with dexfenfluramine in diabetic but not in non-diabetic obese patients (adapted from reference 23).

Interestingly, it was demonstrated that dexfenfluramine partially but significantly corrects these abnormalities in obese diabetic patients, even in the absence of significant weight reduction.[23] In obese patients with type 2 diabetes, basal hepatic glucose output is significantly increased, which contributes to fasting hyperglycaemia despite elevated plasma insulin levels, and suppression of glucose production requires significantly higher delivery rates and plasma concentrations of insulin.[15,21,22] Thus, most obese diabetic patients are characterized by severe insulin resistance at both the hepatic and muscular sites.

One key issue of the presence of insulin resistance in the obese patient with type 2 diabetes is illustrated by the high prevalence of the so-called insulin resistance syndrome, metabolic syndrome or syndrome X.[24,25] Indeed, arterial hypertension, dyslipidaemias, hyperuricaemia, hyperfibrinogenaemia and fibrinolytic disturbances (high PAI-1 levels) are frequently observed in obese diabetic subjects, and particularly in those with high insulin resistance.[26] All these abnormalities markedly increase the cardiovascular risk of such patients.[13,24,25] Consequently, insulin-sensitizing agents, such as thiazolidinediones (glitazones) or metformin, may have practical implications for cardiovascular disease prevention.[27] Insulin resistance and the associated metabolic syndrome are especially linked to abdominal adiposity,[28] so that reduction of visceral fat should be one of the main objectives in the management of the obese diabetic subject.[29]

Several hypotheses have been put forward to explain insulin resistance associated with obesity: schematically they can be divided into a metabolic hypothesis and a haemodynamic hypothesis.

Metabolic hypothesis

Obesity, especially visceral adiposity,[5,28] is associated with increased release and higher plasma levels of free fatty acids (FFA) which may trigger a reduction in insulin sensitivity at both the hepatic and the muscular levels.[30] In the liver, high FFA supply results in an increased glucose output (essentially due to enhanced gluconeogenesis), a decreased insulin extraction and an increased production of 'very-low-density lipoproteins' (VLDL), while in the skeletal muscle such metabolic abnormality results in a reduction in glucose uptake, oxidation and storage as glycogen.[31] Interestingly, muscle biopsy studies have shown a positive relationship between intramyocellular triglyceride content and whole body insulin resistance,[32] and these results were recently confirmed in elegant studies using ^{1}H and ^{13}C nuclear magnetic resonance spectroscopy of skeletal muscle in subjects at high risk of developing type 2 diabetes.[33]

Recent observations, both in animal models and in humans, suggested that tumour necrosis factor-alpha (TNF-α) may play an important role in the insulin resistance associated with excessive adipose mass and be a link between obesity and diabetes.[34] TNF-α is overexpressed in the adipose tissue of obese subjects and could reduce insulin action in the skeletal muscle via a paracrine effect, especially by promoting FFA release from the adipocytes. It is also overexpressed in the muscle itself and a direct negative effect of TNF-α on cellular insulin signalling has been reported.[35] However, while numerous data support the role of TNF-α in rodents, its precise role in human obesity still remains controversial and, until now, the few attempts to block TNF-α failed to improve insulin sensitivity in obese insulin-resistant patients with[36] or without[37] overt type 2 diabetes.

Haemodynamic hypothesis

Besides the metabolic hypothesis attributing a crucial role to FFA and possibly to TNF-α, a haemodynamic hypothesis has also been proposed to explain, at least partially, decreased insulin sensitivity in skeletal muscles.[38,39] Indeed, a reduced skeletal muscle capillary density (in addition to a lower proportion of slow muscle fibres, type 1,), a defective endothelial insulin transport and an impaired insulin-mediated muscular vasodilatation have been reported in obese subjects, especially in those with type 2 diabetes.[38] These abnormalities may limit the diffusion of insulin from the vascular compartment to the target cells, and thus contribute to reduce insulin sensitivity in skeletal muscles.[2,39] Such haemodynamic abnormalities may represent new targets for drugs affecting the vascular tone and improved insulin sensitivity has been reported after treatment with angiotensin converting enzyme inhibitors.[40,41]

Role of insulin secretory defect

Not all obese subjects will become diabetic and only those individuals who are unable to maintain sustained hyperinsulinaemia capable to compensate for insulin resistance are candidates to develop diabetes.[15,42] Several mechanisms have been proposed during the last 10 years to explain such a beta-cell deficiency.[1,2,15] First, a genetic defect may be present, although such a defect has not been detected yet in subjects with common type 2 diabetes associated with obesity. Second, in utero malnutrition may lead to insufficient B cell development and later partial insulin secretory defect (in addition to insulin resistance: 'thrifty phenotype hypothesis'). Third, chronic overstimulation of islet B cell as observed in the early phase of obesity is associated with high secretion of amylin, a peptide which is cosecreted with insulin and can accumulate as amyloid fibrils in pancreatic islets, leading to a progressive impairment of insulin secretion. And fourth, an unfavourable metabolic environment may play a role, especially increased glucose levels which can trigger glucotoxicity,[43] and chronically elevated FFA concentrations which can induce lipotoxicity.[44,45] Indeed, in contrast to an acute rise in FFA levels, which stimulates insulin secretion, chronic elevation of FFA concentrations, a common finding in obese insulin-resistant subjects,[30] rather impairs B cell function.[44,45]

Thus, type 2 diabetes results from a defect in both insulin action and insulin secretion,[46] and these two defects are perpetuated and exaggerated by both lipotoxicity and glucotoxicity in a vicious circle, which may explain the progressive metabolic deterioration generally seen in obese patients with type 2 diabetes (Figure 2.2), a condition which may require frequent adjustments of pharmacological anti-diabetic therapy along with time.[47]

Natural history of diabetes in obese subjects

Type 2 diabetes occurs as a late phenomenon in obese subjects and is preceeded by years of normal glucose tolerance or impaired glucose tolerance (IGT).[15,48,49] The progression from IGT to diabetes occurs when the B cell becomes unable to maintain its previously high rate of insulin secretion in response to glucose. To some extent, the natural history of the obese subjects developing type 2 diabetes may be explained by the 'overworked B cell' hypothesis supported by numerous observations in various animal models.[50] It has recently been reported that long-term changes in insulin action and insulin secretion are associated with gain, loss, regain and maintenance of body weight.[51] Interestingly, weight gain could have more detrimental effects in people with IGT, in whom insulin secretion decreases rather than increases to compensate for the decreased insulin action.

We compared the insulin response to glucose during an OGTT in various groups of obese subjects as a function of fasting blood glucose levels as well as the metabolic clearance rate of glucose measured during a euglycaemic hyperinsulinaemic clamp in obese subjects with various fasting plasma glucose levels. Obese non-diabetic subjects were characterized by a significant reduction in glucose utilization during the clamp, which appeared to be compensated for by an increased insulin response during the OGTT. In contrast, as basal hyperglycaemia increased, there was a progressive decline in glucose metabolic clearance rate (MCR) and simultaneously a dramatic decrease in insulin response during the OGTT.[15] It has been demonstrated that this evolution occurs along the natural history of obesity.[48] During the first years of obesity, the subjects are normoglycaemic but hyperinsulinaemic. Afterwards they become hyperglycaemic at a time when hyperinsulinaemia is no longer maintained.

The authors evaluated insulin secretion, using plasma C peptide levels in the fasting condition and after the intravenous injection of 1 mg glucagon, and insulin sensitivity, by measuring glucose MCR during an euglycaemic hyperinsulinaemic glucose clamp, in six groups of 10 to 15 subjects each (Figure 2.4). These subjects were separated according to the presence or not of obesity (three groups of lean subjects and three groups of obese subjects) and according to the presence or not of diabetes (two groups with normal glucose tolerance, two groups with non insulin-requiring type 2 diabetes and two groups with insulin-requiring diabetes, one group of lean subjects and one group of obese subjects in each category).[15] Obese patients with normal glucose tolerance were characterized by a significant reduction in insulin sensitivity, which was almost fully compensated for by an appropriate increase in insulin secretion. Obese patients with non-insulin-requiring diabetes showed an even lower insulin sensitivity which was associated with a partial

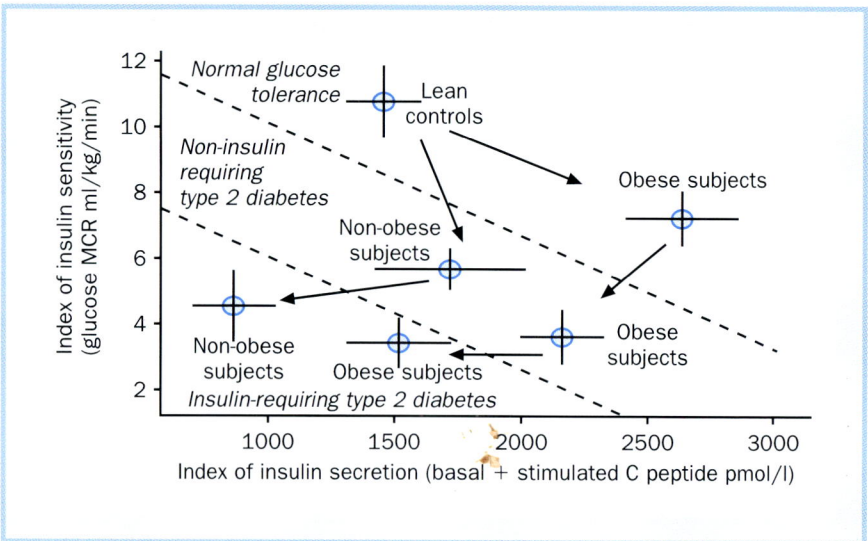

Figure 2.4
Hypothetical scheme of the natural history of type 2 diabetes mellitus: changes in insulin secretion and insulin sensitivity in six groups of 10 to 15 subjects, three without obesity ('lean') and three with obesity ('obese'). The upper broken line separates non-diabetic subjects (with normal glucose tolerance) and non-insulin-requiring diabetic patients, while the lower broken line separates non-insulin-requiring and insulin-requiring diabetic patients. Results are expressed as mean ± SEM (from reference 15).

defect in insulin secretion. Finally, obese patients with insulin-requiring type 2 diabetes were characterized by a marked reduction in insulin secretion without further worsening of insulin resistance. In the absence of obesity, the same progression of endocrine abnormalities was observed according to the severity of diabetes, but each group of lean subjects was characterized by a lower insulin secretion rate and, in most cases, a better insulin sensitivity than the corresponding group of obese subjects (Figure 2.4).

Thus, type 2 diabetes occurs when obese subjects can no longer maintain hyperinsulinaemia to compensate for decreased insulin sensitivity and late progression to the insulin-requiring state is best explained by an exhaustion of insulin secretion in the face of persistent severe insulin resistance.[52]

Reversibility of diabetes after marked weight loss in obese subjects

While the natural history of the progression from obesity to diabetes is well depicted,[15;48] it is interesting to consider the reverse way and to investigate whether weight loss in severely obese subjects is able to prevent diabetes, to help in the treatment of the disease or even to suppress hyperglycaemia and associated metabolic risk factors.[9,10]

A substantial and sustained weight loss can be obtained after bariatric surgery in subjects with severe/extreme obesity.[53] Post-gastroplasty recovery of ideal body weight resulted in a complete normalization of insulin action, insulin clearance and insulin secretion in severely obese, non-diabetic patients.[54] Such beneficial effects may explain why weight loss drastically decreases the incidence of type 2 diabetes in such a population.[3;9] In addition, we showed in a large cohort of non-diabetic obese subjects that post-gastroplasty weight loss was associated with a remarkable correction of all metabolic markers associated with the insulin resistance syndrome.[55] As all these markers are considered as cardiovascular risk factors,[24–26] such favourable effects will probably result in a significant improvement in the cardiovascular prognosis of obese patients.[13] Both biological and histological markers of non-alcoholic steatohepatitis (NASH), which were present in most severely obese patients, also regressed after weight loss, in a manner parallel to the classical markers of the insulin resistance syndrome.[56] Finally, we reported that blood glucose control of obese patients with type 2 diabetes was markedly improved after a sustained weight loss following gastroplasty, allowing a remarkable reduction in the doses of hypoglycaemic agents (see below).[9,10,53]

Thus, the progression from normal glucose tolerance to IGT and type 2 diabetes seen in numerous obese subjects can be reversed by a substantial and sustained weight loss, a condition which also remarkably improves blood glucose control in patients with overt diabetes. Thus, all efforts should be made to promote weight loss in obese patients with type 2 diabetes or in subjects at risk of developing the disease.[57,58]

Dietary regimen and very-low-calorie diets

Medical nutrition therapy is an essential component of successful diabetes management.[59,60] The three main goals in the dietary management of obese diabetic patients are.

(1)   To achieve and maintain a reasonable body weight;
(2)   To keep blood glucose levels in as near-normal range as possible; and
(3)   To achieve optimal lipid levels.

A daily energy deficit of 500–1000 kcal mobilizes fat preferentially and causes 0.5–1.0 kg weight loss per week. However, achieving and maintaining weight loss may be difficult for the obese patient, essentially because of poor compliance to long-term restricted diet. Moreover, weight loss is less impressive in obese diabetic versus non-diabetic subjects, probably because the improvement of glucose control associated with weight reduction results

in less glycosuria and thus less caloric loss.[61] Consequently, rather than encouraging obese diabetic patients to reach ideal or desirable weights, reasonable weight goals should be determined. Several studies have indeed demonstrated that a modest weight loss can already improve the metabolic control of obese diabetic patients, at least in the short term (reviewed in references 62 and 63); however, only a major weight reduction is most likely to reverse hyperglycaemia in the long term (reviewed in references 9 and 10). Several studies have reported favourable effects of weight loss induced by low-calorie diets,[58,64,65] although such effects may be transient due to only short-lasting weight reduction. Very-low-calorie diets (VLCDs) provide 400–800 kcal/day of high-quality protein and carbohydrate fortified with vitamins, minerals and trace elements. Several studies indicated that VLCDs are safe for use by obese diabetic patients in a medical setting closely supervised by an experienced physician and that the numerous metabolic benefits derived from VLCD therapy outweigh its risk.[58,64,65] Improvement in glycaemic control occurs quickly, resulting from increased insulin action in the liver and peripheral tissues, and enhanced insulin secretion. It occurs with only modest weight reduction, suggesting that caloric restriction plays a more critical role, at least initially. The conclusions of a recent meta-analysis of 89 studies involving 1800 subjects were that dietary strategies are most effective for promoting short-term weight loss in type 2 diabetes.[58] Dieting, especially by VLCD, is a very effective way to lose between 5 and 10 kg weight, and consequently to improve glycated haemoglobin (HbA_{1c}) levels. However, in most studies, some data were incomplete concerning the description of subjects, interventions or longitudinal outcomes beyond 12 months after intervention.

Anti-obesity pharmacotherapy in the management of type 2 diabetes

Weight reduction should be considered as a key objective in the management of the obese diabetic patient (Figure 2.5). In this respect,

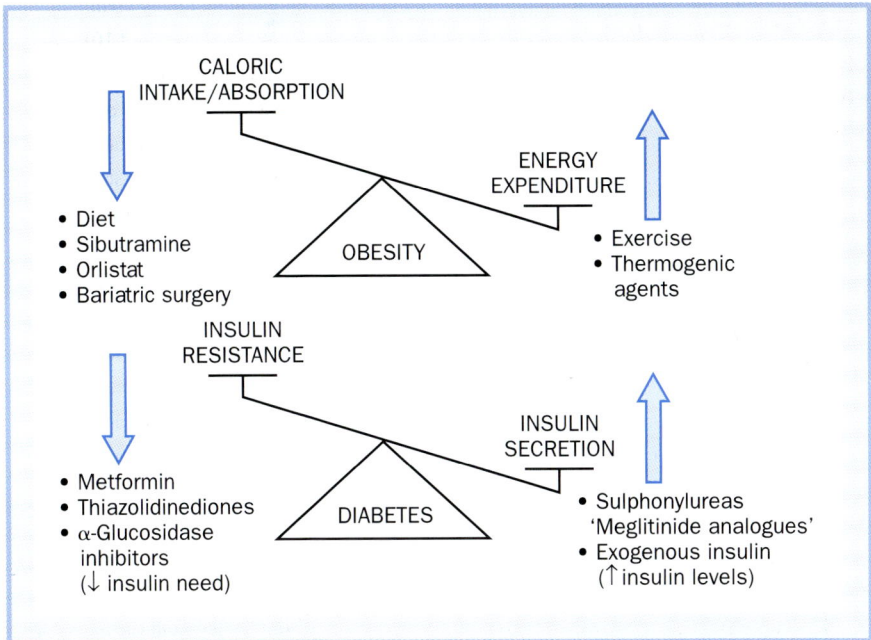

Figure 2.5
Strategies targeting either obesity (reduction of caloric intake/absorption and/or stimulation of energy expenditure) or diabetes (reduction of insulin resistance and/or stimulation of insulin secretion) for the management of obese diabetic patients (from reference 12).

several anti-obesity drugs have demonstrated a potential interest.[66–68] However, while fenfluramine and dexfenfluramine have been shown to promote weight loss and to improve insulin sensitivity directly,[23] two mechanisms contributing to a better blood glucose control in obese type 2 diabetic patients (reviewed in references 10 and 11), they were recently withdrawn because of safety problems.[67,68] Benfluorex, which is structurally related to fenfluramine, is a known hypolipidaemic agent with possible glucose-lowering effects, especially in the obese diabetic patient, despite the absence of significant effect on body weight (reviewed references in 69 and 70). It has been shown to improve glucose tolerance and metabolic control in obese individuals with type 2 diabetes on a body-weight-maintaining diet by increasing sensitivity to insulin without directly stimulating insulin secretion.[71–73] Two recent double-blind, placebo-controlled trials showed that benfluorex potentiates the effects of a hypocaloric diet on weight loss and on glycaemic control in obese type 2 diabetic patients treated with insulin, presumably by increasing insulin sensitivity.[74,75]

Other novel pharmacological approaches deserve further consideration, for instance beta-3 agonists aiming to increase energy expenditure, drugs interfering with TNF-α or FFA release by the adipose tissue or agents slowing gastric emptying (Figure 2.5) (reviewed in reference 11). However, until

now, results regarding efficacy and/or safety are disappointing or only preliminary in humans. Thus, in the present review, we will focus only on the potential efficacy in the management of obese diabetic patients of two recently marketed anti-obesity agents: sibutramine, a new selective norepinephrine and serotonin reuptake inhibitor, and orlistat, a selective gastrointestinal lipase inhibitor.

Sibutramine

Sibutramine has been shown to produce a dose-related weight loss in obese subjects, at optimal doses of 10–20 mg/day.[76,77] This effect results predominantly from a significant reduction in food intake. An early study in obese patients with type 2 diabetes treated with a variety of hypoglycaemic agents suggested that weight loss following therapy with sibutramine resulted in improved glycaemic control (Table 2.1).[78] In diet-treated obese patients with type 2 diabetes, sibutramine-induced weight loss was accompanied by a shift towards improved metabolic control (lower HbA_{1c} levels) and the reduction in fasting plasma glucose was proportional to the degree of weight loss.[76,79–84] Similar favourable results were recently reported in obese, sulphonylurea-treated[85] or metformin-treated[86] type 2 diabetic patients (Table 2.1). In all studies, the differences versus placebo were more pronounced and statistically significant in so-

Table 2.1
Effects of sibutramine on blood glucose control in obese patients with type 2 diabetes in placebo-controlled, double-blind, parallel clinical trials. All studies were reported in international congresses and published as abstracts only, except the study of Finer et al.[78] Results are expressed as changes versus placebo.

Reference	Usual anti-diabetic treatment	Dose of sibutramine (mg/day)	Sibutramine/ placebo (n)	Trial duration (weeks)	Body weight loss (kg)	Fasting plasma glucose (mmol/l)	HbA$_{1c}$ %
Vargas et al[79]	NA	20	9/9	12	−2.2	−0.7	NA
Griffiths et al[80]	Various	15	45/46	12	−2.3	−0.2	−0.40
Fujioka et al[81]	Various	20	89/86	24	−4.0	−1.3[a]	−0.53[a]
Peirce et al[82]	Diet alone	15	18/17	12	−0.9	NA	−0.20
Rissanen[83] Heath et al[84]	Diet alone	15	114/122	52	−4.5	−0.2	−0.10
Serrano-Rios et al[85]	Sulphonylurea	15 or 20	131/65	24	−3.0	NA	−0.40[b]
McNulty et al[86]	Metformin	15 or 20	NA/NA	52	−6.5	NA	−0.22 (−0.95[a])
Finer et al[78]	Various	15	47/44	12	−2.3	−1.7	−0.30

NA: not available in the abstract reporting the trial.
[a] placebo versus ≥5% weight loss sibutramine responders.
[b] placebo versus ≥10% weight loss sibutramine responders.

called sibutramine responders, i.e. patients losing ≥5% or ≥10% of initial body weight. Improvement of lipid profile after sibutramine-induced weight loss was also observed in three placebo-controlled randomized trials[87] while the effect on arterial blood pressure was almost negligible.

A meta-analysis of placebo-controlled studies performed in modestly hyperglycaemic obese patients showed that greater improvements in fasting plasma glucose concentrations were observed in the group receiving sibutramine.[88] This difference was probably explained by the fact that more patients (almost double) on sibutramine rather than on placebo achieved significant weight loss; the observation that changes in plasma glucose levels observed on sibutramine and placebo were similar for the same degree of weight loss indeed suggests an indirect rather than a direct action of the drug on glucose metabolism. One study using the hyperinsulinaemic clamp demonstrated a similar improvement in insulin sensitivity in obese type 2 diabetic patients after a comparable weight loss of about 5 kg obtained with either sibutramine or placebo.[82] Thus, in contrast to the observations previously reported with dexfenfluramine and fluoxetine (reviewed in references 10 and 11), no improvement in insulin sensitivity has been demonstrated with sibutramine independent of weight loss.

In a French multicentre study performed in obese patients at risk of developing diabetes, sibutramine resulted in significantly greater weight loss and improved glucose tolerance.[89] Finally, the Sibutramine Trial of Obesity Reduction and Maintenance (STORM) is a recent multicentre study evaluating weight loss and weight maintenance with sibutramine 10 mg once daily.[90] In 505 of 605 obese non-diabetic patients completing the first 6-month open-label phase of the study, sibutramine in addition to diet resulted in mean reductions in body weight of −11.3 kg, in waist circumference of −9.7 cm, in HbA_{1c} of −0.3%, in fasting glucose of −0.15 mmol/l and in insulin of −10.4 pmol/l; again, these changes were more marked in those patients losing 5 or 10% of baseline body weight. The changes observed in the subsequent 18-month, placebo-controlled, double-blind weight maintenance phase demonstrated sustained metabolic improvement in the sibutramine group but not the placebo group.[91] These promising results should encourage further long-term studies with sibutramine in obese patients with type 2 diabetes.

Orlistat

Orlistat, a semisynthetic derivative of lipstatin, is a potent and selective inhibitor of gastric and pancreatic lipases.[92] When administered with fat-containing foods, it partially inhibits the hydrolysis of triglycerides, thus reducing the subsequent absorption of monoglycerides and free fatty acids. Orlistat treatment resulted in a dose-dependent reduction in body weight of obese subjects, with an optimal dosage regimen of 120 mg tid, and was well tolerated with the exception of mild-to-moderate and transient gastrointestinal events.[93] Orlistat is the anti-obesity compound which has been well evaluated in placebo-controlled, long-term studies involving large number of patients. In several 1–2-year trials,[94–97] orlistat, when used with a health-promoting low-fat and moderately energy-restricted diet, induced significantly greater weight loss and better weight maintenance, with a specific reduction in total and LDL cholesterol serum levels as compared to placebo. Concomitant reductions in plasma glucose and insulin levels were also reported, and this effect is probably due to the weight loss induced by orlistat, rather than a direct effect of the drug on insulin sensitivity.

An analysis of pooled data from US and European placebo-controlled clinical trials involving 675 obese subjects compared oral glucose tolerance tests (OGTTs) before and after 104 weeks of follow-up. The results showed that:

(1) A smaller percentage of subjects with IGT at baseline progressed to diabetic status in the orlistat (3.0%) versus placebo (7.6%) group;

(2) Conversely, among subjects with IGT at baseline, glucose levels normalized in more subjects after orlistat treatment (71.6%) versus placebo (49.1%); and

(3) In patients with criteria of diabetes at baseline, more patients reverted to IGT or normal values during the OGTT after orlistat (57.9%) than after placebo (28.6%)[98] (Figure 2.6).

These results suggest that orlistat may assist in reducing the deterioration of glucose tolerance among those obese individuals most at risk for the development of diabetes mellitus, and may even help in reverting IGT or mild type 2 diabetes as already suggested in some preliminary published work (reviewed in reference 11).

A large multicentre, randomized, double-blind, placebo-controlled study was undertaken to determine the effects of orlistat (3×120 mg/day) in obese type 2 diabetic patients treated with oral hypoglycaemic agents.[99] After 1 year of treatment, a mean difference of 2.4 kg weight reduction was observed in the orlistat group versus the placebo group and twice as many patients receiving orlistat lost ≥5% of initial body weight (49 versus 23%, $P < 0.001$). Such modest weight loss was associated with significant differences in fasting plasma glucose (-0.56 mmol/l) and HbA$_{1c}$ (-0.45%) levels (Figure 2.6). Furthermore, a significant reduction in the dose of sulphonylureas was seen in the orlistat group (-23% versus -9% with placebo, $P < 0.002$) as well as a clear-cut improvement in lipid parameters, with significantly greater reductions in total

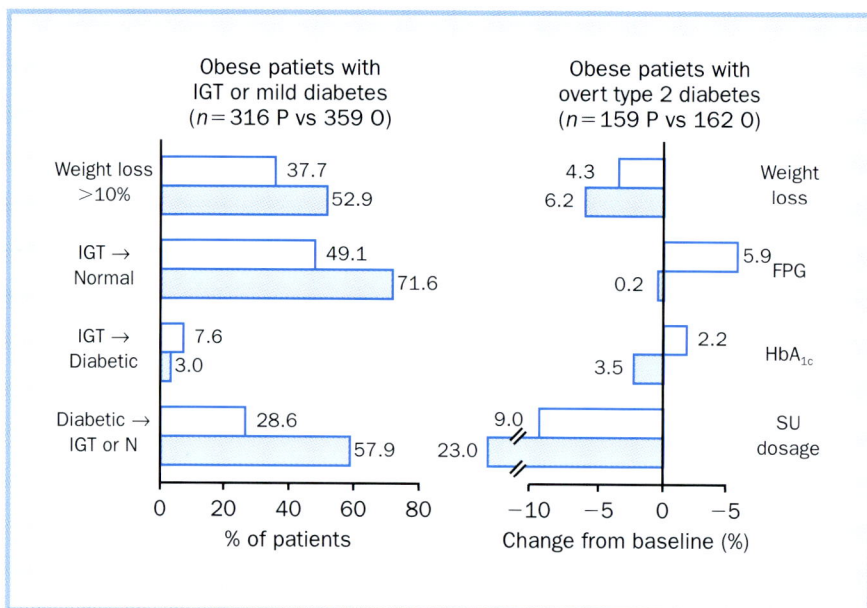

Figure 2.6
Effects of orlistat (O, hatched columns) versus placebo (P, open columns) on glucose tolerance assessed during an oral glucose tolerance test in obese subjects at risk of developing diabetes (left panel, adapted from reference 98) and on blood glucose control in obese patients with type 2 diabetes treated with diet and sulphonylureas (SU) (right panel, adapted from reference 97). All differences between orlistat and placebo were statistically significant. IGT: impaired glucose tolerance, N: normal glucose tolerance, FPG: fasting plasma glucose.

cholesterol, LDL cholesterol, triglycerides, apolipoprotein B and LDL to HDL cholesterol ratio as compared to placebo (all $P < 0.001$ except, $P < 0.05$ for triglycerides). While the effects on blood glucose control appear to be fully explained by the modest orlistat-associated weight loss, the impact of orlistat on several lipid parameters was independent of the magnitude of weight reduction and should be

related to the mechanism of action by reducing the absorption of dietary fat. Thus, this study demonstrated that orlistat is an effective treatment modality in obese patients with type 2 diabetes with respect to clinically meaningful weight loss and maintenance of weight loss, improved glycaemic control and improved lipid profile.[99]

Finally, two recent meta-analyses of five

multicentre randomized, placebo-controlled trials suggested that orlistat-associated weight loss resulted in a significant reduction in insulin resistance,[100] and that orlistat treatment may be of particular benefit in reducing coronary heart disease risk for abdominally obese dyslipidaemic patients.[101] These favourable effects on the cardiovascular risk profile of non-diabetic obese patients[102] may be particularly important in obese patients with type 2 diabetes whose cardiovascular risk is known to be markedly increased.[103]

Anti-diabetic agents in the management of the obese diabetic patient

Four pharmacological classes of oral agents are currently used for treating type 2 diabetes: sulphonylureas (or more recently new insulin secretagogues of the meglitinide family), biguanides (metformin), α-glucosidase inhibitors (acarbose and miglitol) and thiazolidinediones, also called glitazones (troglitazone which has been recently withdrawn because of hepatotoxicity, rosiglitazone and pioglitazone)[104,105] (Figure 2.7). If the oral treatment fails, insulin therapy may be prescribed, alone or in combination with oral agents. The selection of an oral anti-diabetic compound depends on several factors, including the severity of hyperglycaemia and some characteristics of the patient, especially the presence of obesity.[11,106]

Sulphonylureas and other insulin secretagogues

The oral administration of drugs which aim at stimulating insulin release (in clinical practice, sulphonylureas or in some countries, meglitinide analogues such as repaglinide or nateglinide) is a cornerstone in the treatment of type 2 diabetes.[107,108] However, such an approach may be less relevant in the obese diabetic patient.[10] Those who oppose the use of sulphonylureas often argue that sulphonylurea treatment could be counterproductive because it may lead to weight gain, hyperinsulinaemia and even more severe insulin resistance, all effects which are particularly unwanted in obese subjects. It is essential that this series of events be kept in mind whenever sulphonylurea therapy is started and that every effort is made to prevent it. In the United Kingdom Prospective Diabetes Study (UKPDS), sulphonylurea therapy with either chlorpropamide or glibenclamide in overweight patients with newly diagnosed type 2 diabetes that could not be controlled with diet therapy resulted in an average 3.7 kg weight gain after 6 years.[109]

The main indications for the use of sulphonylureas in obese diabetic patients are:

(1) When rather severe hyperglycaemia is present;

(2) When monotherapy with metformin does not achieve adequate glycaemic control;

(3) When metformin is contra-indicated or not well tolerated; and possibly

(4) In combination with bedtime insulin after secondary failure to oral agents (see below).

Metformin

Since its early use in Europe, the biguanide compound metformin has been more particularly recommended in obese rather than non-obese type 2 diabetic patients.[106] Indeed, the drug lowers plasma glucose levels without increasing (and even by concomitantly decreasing) circulating insulin concentrations, suggesting that it may improve insulin sensitivity.[110] The United Kingdom Prospective Diabetes Study (UKPDS) recently demonstrated, in obese subjects with newly diagnosed type 2 diabetes, that metformin monotherapy was associated with a significant reduction in diabetes-related complications and cardiovascular morbidity when compared with diet alone or even with intensive therapy using sulphonylureas or insulin.[111] In addition, this study clearly showed that, despite a similar improvement in blood glucose control, weight gain was significantly less pronounced with metformin than with sulphonylureas or insulin. The mechanisms for such a difference remain unclear. However, two recent studies demonstrated that metformin therapy was associated with a significant reduction in food intake in obese non-diabetic subjects[112] and in insulin-treated obese diabetic patients.[113] The latter study also showed that metformin prevents weight gain in type 2 diabetic patients receiving exogenous insulin. Thus, such an anorectic effect of metformin represents a further argument to consider the biguanide compound as a first choice anti-diabetic agent in obese patients with type 2 diabetes.[106] Finally, the ongoing Diabetes Prevention Program, involving 27 clinical centres in the USA and recruiting at least 3000 participants, will test the possibility of preventing or delaying the onset of type 2 diabetes (and, as secondary endpoint, cardiovascular complications) with metformin versus placebo in individuals at high risk, selected on the basis of weight excess (BMI ≥ 24 kg/m^2) and criteria of IGT during an OGTT.[114]

α-Glucosidase inhibitors

α-Glucosidase inhibitors (acarbose, miglitol and voglibose) exert a competitive, dose-dependent, inhibition of small intestinal α-glucosidase enzymes which break down non-absorbable complex carbohydrates into absorbable monosaccharides.[115] At doses tolerated by man, energy loss is not significant and weight reduction not attained.[115–117] However, such a pharmacological action leads to a delayed and reduced rise in post-prandial blood glucose levels, and consequently plasma insulin concentrations, an effect which may be particularly appreciated in obese diabetic patients. Several studies have shown that acarbose improves indices of blood glucose stability in type 2 diabetic subjects treated with diet, oral hypoglycaemic agents or insulin.[115–118] Reductions of HbA_{1C} levels by about 0.6–0.7% were obtained without increasing, or even reducing, body weight and the incidence of hypoglycaemic episodes. The UKPDS group recently demonstrated on a large cohort of type 2 diabetic patients that such a favourable effect of acarbose on glycaemic control persisted up to 3 years, with no significant difference in body weight.[119]

Even without inducing a significant weight loss, α-glucosidase inhibitors may represent a useful adjunct therapy for the obese diabetic patient insufficiently controlled by diet alone or in combination with other classical anti-diabetic drugs.

Thiazolidinediones

Thiazolidinediones or glitazones (troglitazone, rosiglitazone, pioglitazone, etc) are a new class of pharmacological compounds which work by enhancing insulin action ('insulin sensitizers') and thus promoting glucose utilization in peripheral tissues and suppressing gluconeogenesis in the liver.[120,121] As agonists of 'peroxisome proliferator activated receptor' or PPAR-γ, a member of the nuclear hormone receptor superfamily,

they enhance the expression of a number of genes encoding proteins involved in glucose and lipid metabolism.[121] Thiazolidinediones stimulate adipogenesis and reduce plasma triglyceride and FFA concentrations. Stimulation of PPAR-γ may decrease the release by the adipocytes of various signalling molecules, such as FFA, leptin, resistin and TNF-α, which are all able to counteract the hypoglycaemic action of insulin.[120,121] Numerous studies have demonstrated that thiazolidinediones improve blood glucose control in (obese) type 2 diabetic patients, treated either by diet alone, or with sulphonylureas, metformin or insulin.[122,123] However, several clinical trials have also reported a mild, although significant, weight gain in type 2 diabetic patients treated with troglitazone, rosiglitazone or pioglitazone for several months.[122,123] The mechanisms responsible for such a weight gain remain poorly understood, but troglitazone has been shown to reduce plasma leptin concentrations and increase hunger in poorly controlled type 2 diabetic patients.[124] Thus, although such a pharmacological approach may be interesting in obese diabetic subjects because of its favourable action on insulin sensitivity, glucose control and other vascular risk factors,[123] interest in its clinical effect might decrease if long-term studies confirm that it promotes weight gain.[122] In addition, the clinical use of compounds of this family may be limited because of safety problems.

Insulin

When insulin secretion becomes insufficient to compensate for insulin resistance, administration of exogenous insulin may be the only solution to protect against severe hyperglycaemia[125–127] (Figure 2.5). However, even if insulin can improve glycaemic control, it is rarely effective in achieving tight glycaemic control, despite increases in resource use.[128] In addition, high doses are usually required in obese diabetic patients, and there is a risk of a substantial increase in body weight, unless there is good dietary compliance.[129] The mechanisms involved may include reduced energy loss through glycosuria, undetected mild hypoglycaemia, primary stimulation of appetite, enhancement of lipogenesis and a reduction in some components of energy expenditure (reviewed in reference 125).

The results from the UKPDS[109] showed that the weight increase during insulin therapy averaged 10.4 kg after 6 years of follow-up in a primary diet failure group of obese patients with newly diagnosed type 2 diabetes. Most of the weight gain occurred during the first year, with a slower gain during subsequent years. In studies in patients with type 2 diabetes and secondary failure to oral agents, insulin administration for 3–12 months produced average weight gains of up to 6 kg (reviewed in reference 125). A recent analysis of 100 insulin-treated type 2 diabetic patients in the Finnish Multicentre Insulin Therapy Study concluded that:

(1) After an initial good response, glycaemic control deteriorates more in obese than in non-obese patients;

(2) In obese patients, weight gain per se cannot explain the poor glycaemic response to insulin therapy, but it may induce a disproportionately large increase in insulin requirements because of greater insulin resistance in the obese than in the non-obese group; and

(3) Weight gain appears harmful as it is associated with increases in blood pressure and low density lipoprotein cholesterol levels.[129]

Consequently, the place of insulin therapy, especially when excessive dosages are required, remains controversial in the management of the obese diabetic patient.[130,131]

Combined therapy

As type 2 diabetes is a heterogenous disease with multiple metabolic and hormonal abnormalities, especially when associated with obesity,[1] it appears logical to combine drug therapies in order to have a positive impact on various sites[104,105,132] (Figure 2.7). Several placebo-controlled studies have investigated the effects of combining insulin with either sulphonylureas, metformin, acarbose or glitazones. The most studied combination comprises NPH insulin at bedtime and sulphonylureas before each main meal. It has been shown that such a regimen provides the best glycaemic control with the least weight gain, as compared to insulin twice daily or multiple insulin injections per day.[133] A recent meta-analysis of 16 studies showed that combination therapy may be a more appropriate and a suitable option to insulin monotherapy in subjects with type 2 diabetes in whom failure to sulphonylurea

developed;[134] most of the subjects included in these studies were, however, only slightly overweight (on average, 112% of ideal body weight). In obese insulin-resistant diabetic patients, it may be interesting to combine other oral anti-diabetic agents with insulin. Favourable results with decreases in blood glucose and HbA_{1c} levels despite a significant reduction in daily insulin dosage have been reported with metformin,[135–137] troglitazone[138] or acarbose.[139] As recently pointed out,[113]

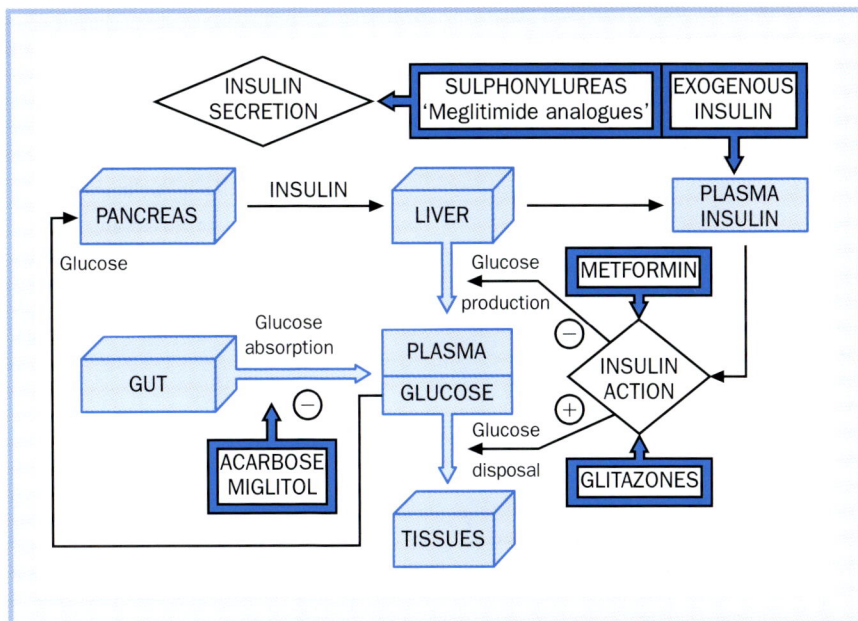

Figure 2.7
Current status of drug treatment of type 2 diabetes: sites of action of sulphonylureas (or 'meglitinide analogues' agents such as repaglinide or nateglinide), metformin, α-glucosidase inhibitors (acarbose, miglitol), thiazolidinediones (glitazones) and exogenous insulin. + = stimulation; − = inhibition (adapted from reference 106).

metformin should be considered as a valuable adjunct to insulin therapy in type 2 diabetic patients with initial overweight or progressive weight gain with insulin.

Bariatric surgery for treating severely obese diabetic patients

The crucial contribution of weight excess to hyperglycaemia in the obese diabetic patient justifies that aggressive weight reduction strategies may be considered in well-selected individuals with refractory obesity and persistent hyperglycaemia despite classical medical approaches[9] (Figures 2.1 and 2.5). According to the NIH consensus development conference,[140] 'patients whose body mass index (BMI) exceeds 40 are potential candidates for surgery and, in certain instances, less severely obese patients (with BMIs between 36 and 41) also may be considered for surgery (included in this category are patients with . . . severe diabetes mellitus)'. It was also mentioned that 'weight reduction surgery has been reported to improve several comorbid conditions such as . . . glucose intolerance and frank diabetes mellitus'. Bariatric surgery indeed prevents the progression of IGT to diabetes.[141] Preliminary results of the large prospective controlled 'Swedish Obese Subjects' study, obtained 2 years after gastroplasty-associated weight loss, demonstrated a marked reduction of the incidence of diabetes which fell down to near zero: the adjusted odds ratio for the surgically treated group versus controls was 0.02, with 95% CI 0.00, 0.16.[142] Furthermore, it has been reported that bariatric surgery allows a remarkable lowering of hyperglycaemia in patients with overt type 2 diabetes and the suppression or at least drastic reduction of anti-diabetic drugs, especially insulin and sulphonylureas (reviewed in references 9 and 10). These favourable effects may be so impressive that Pories and coworkers claimed that type 2 diabetes may be considered a surgical disease,[143] and that an operation is the most effective therapy for adult-onset diabetes mellitus.[144] Among all proposed surgical procedures, it appears that techniques leading to a gastric restriction (vertical gastroplasty, silicone adjustable gastric banding) or gastric bypass have the most favourable benefit to risk ratio.[53,145]

Our group studied 31 severely obese patients with overt diabetes mellitus in whom a vertical ring gastroplasty was performed resulting in a marked weight reduction of about 30 kg (Table 2.2). Despite the fact that body weight was not normalized, a remarkable improvement in the glycaemic control was observed which persisted more than 2 years after surgery. This metabolic improvement was observed despite a marked diminution of the anti-diabetic treatment. In addition to the improvement of glycaemic control, gastroplasty-induced weight loss resulted in a clear-cut reduction of other risk factors such as arterial hypertension and dyslipidaemias (Table 2.2).

The ultimate objective of bariatric surgery is not to reduce risk factors but to improve the prognosis and the quality of life of the obese patient. No prospective study has demonstrated that bariatric surgery prolongs life expectancy when compared to medical supervision, especially in the population with type 2 diabetes. Nevertheless, a pilot study compared the outcome of 154 obese diabetic subjects submitted to gastric bypass with that of 78 obese subjects who were not submitted to surgery (used as controls).[146] After a mean follow-up of 6.2 years and 9 years,

respectively, the mortality rate in the control group was 28%, compared to 9% in the surgical group (including perioperative deaths) ($P < 0.0003$). For every year of follow-up, patients in the control group had a 4.5% chance of dying versus a 1.0% chance for those in the surgical group ($P < 0.0001$). This improvement in the mortality rate in the surgical group was primarily due to a decrease in the number of cardiovascular deaths. Such favourable results, which are in agreement with the remarkable reduction in risk factors, should be verified in a larger prospective study such as the ongoing Swedish Obese Subjects study.[142]

Table 2.2
Body mass index (BMI), blood glucose control, arterial blood pressure and lipid profile in 31 obese type 2 diabetic patients before and 24 ± 7 months after gastroplasty.

	Before gastroplasty	After gastroplasty	P
BMI (kg/m^2)	44.4 ± 1.3	33.6 ± 0.9	0.001
Fasting plasma glucose (mmol/l)	9.00 ± 0.67	6.06 ± 0.39	0.001
HbA_{1c} (%)	8.2 ± 0.4	5.8 ± 0.3	0.003
Systolic blood pressure (mm Hg)	162 ± 40	137 ± 40	0.001
Diastolic blood pressure (mm Hg)	94 ± 20	79 ± 20	0.001
Triglycerides (mg/dl)	208 ± 19	147 ± 22	0.04
Total cholesterol (mg/dl)	231 ± 9	227 ± 12	NS
HDL cholesterol (mg/dl)	43 ± 4	48 ± 5	0.03
LDL cholesterol (mg/dl)	150 ± 7	170 ± 11	NS

Note: Anti-diabetic treatment (after versus before gastroplasty: 2 versus 8 patients on sulphonylureas, 7 versus 21 on metformin and 5 versus 8 on insulin) and anti-hypertensive therapy could be reduced or stopped in most patients after weight loss.

Overall management of the obese diabetic patient

The management of the obese diabetic patient remains a challenge for the clinician (Figure 2.8). Strategies include:

(1) Promoting weight loss, through the use of lifestyle modifications (hypocaloric diet and exercise), very-low-calorie diets, anti-obesity drugs and even, in well-selected cases, bariatric surgery;

(2) Improving glycaemic control, through a reduction in insulin resistance (lifestyle modifications, metformin, insulin sensitizers such as thiazolidinediones, benfluorex), a correction of insulinopenia

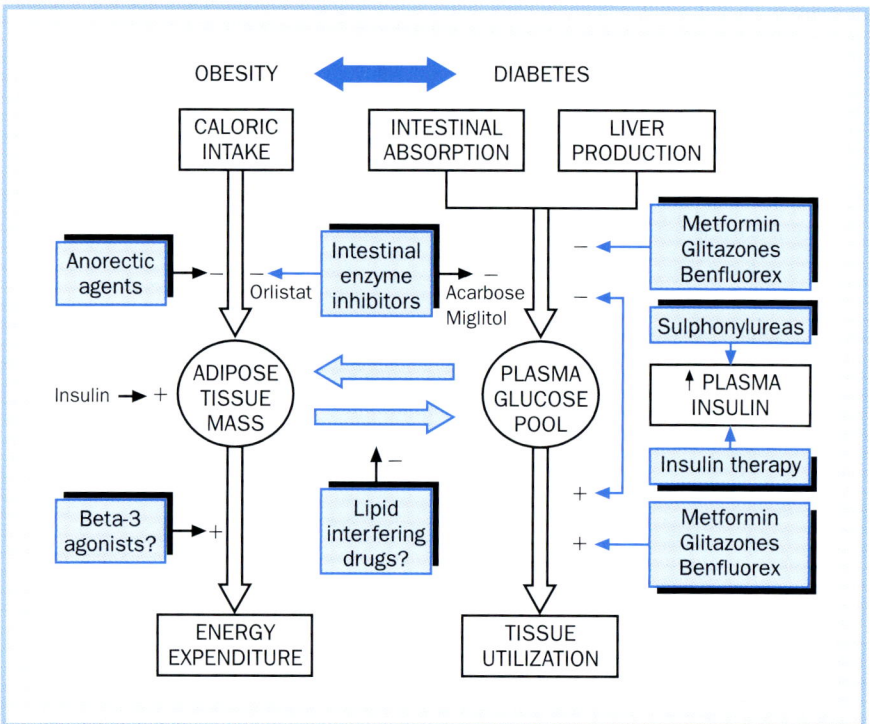

Figure 2.8
Integrated scheme illustrating the sites of action of the main drugs used in the treatment of the obese diabetic patient. + = stimulation; − = inhibition. Beta-3 agonists and lipid-interfering drugs are still in clinical development (adapted from reference 10).

(insulin secretagogues, for example, sulphonylureas, or exogenous insulin) and/or a delay in carbohydrate intestinal absorption (acarbose); and/or

(3) Treating associated risk factors, such as arterial hypertension and dyslipidaemias, to improve the cardiovascular prognosis (Figure 2.1) (reviewed in reference 10).

It should be noted, however, that the improvement in glycaemic control may limit weight reduction, and even promote weight gain and worsen other risk factors. In the obese diabetic individual, anti-diabetic agent selection should favour compounds which improve insulin action rather than those which stimulate insulin secretion. Exogenous insulin alone is rarely successful in obese diabetic patients so that combined therapy is often preferable, especially with metformin.

When morbid obesity is present, both restoration of good glycaemic control and correction of associated risk factors can only be obtained through a drastic weight loss. This primary objective justifies more aggressive weight reduction programmes in well-selected individuals. New anti-obesity drugs, such as sibutramine and orlistat, may provide an additional approach for the treatment of type 2 diabetes, although available data suggest that the overall efficacy on body weight and glycaemic control is generally modest. Thus, treatment with sibutramine or orlistat should be reserved for those patients who, for still unknown reasons, are good responders to such a therapy, that is those who are capable of obtaining and maintaining a $\geq 5\%$ loss of initial body weight. Finally, in massively obese subjects (BMI >40 kg/m^2 or >35 kg/m^2 with severe comorbidities), remarkable results have been reported with bariatric surgery with, in most cases, an alleviation or even a complete cure of diabetes mellitus. However, such a surgical procedure should only be performed by a well-trained multidisciplinary team in well-selected and carefully supervised patients.

Conclusions

The evolution from obesity to diabetes represents a continuum that progresses through different phases in which defects in both insulin action and insulin secretion play a critical interaction and must be looked at in concert. The improved knowledge of the natural history of type 2 diabetes associated with obesity may have important therapeutic implications. Pharmacological efforts are focused on drugs that increase insulin sensitivity and/or drugs that preserve B cell function. However, it is obvious that the most effective way to improve the prognosis of obese patients is to obtain sustained weight loss. Further studies are necessary to improve the identification of good responders to pharmacotherapy and to specify the role of anti-obesity agents in the overall long-term management of obese subjects with type 2 diabetes.

The management of the obese diabetic patient should combine strategies which aim at reducing weight excess, lowering chronic hyperglycaemia and correcting other risk factors. Weight loss is a major target in treating obese patients with type 2 diabetes as it allows simultaneous improvement in both glycaemic control and associated risk factors, whereas specific anti-hyperglycaemic treatment, with sulphonylureas or insulin (but not metformin), usually favours weight gain and may worsen the risk profile. Aggressive weight reduction programmes may be used in severely obese individuals with type 2 diabetes, refractory to conventional diet and drug treatment. In particular, bariatric surgery may be helpful in diabetic subjects with morbid obesity. However, even if weight loss appears to be the cornerstone of successful treatment, long-term prospective studies are still required to determine more precisely the place of each strategy in the overall management of obese diabetic patients (evidence-based medicine). Obviously, the prevention of obesity should be considered a key objective by medical practitioners and public health authorities in order to limit the expected epidemic of type 2 diabetes mellitus in this early new millennium.

References

1   Scheen AJ, Lefèbvre PJ, Pathophysiology of type 2 diabetes. In: Kuhlmann J, Puls W, eds, *Handbook of Experimental Pharmacology, Oral Antidiabetics* (Springer Verlag: Berlin, 1996) 7–42.

2   DeFronzo RA, Pathogenesis of type 2 diabetes: metabolic and molecular implications for identifying diabetes genes, *Diabetes Rev* (1997) **5**:177–269.

3   Pi-Sunyer FX, Weight and non-insulin-dependent diabetes mellitus, *Am J Clin Nutr* (1996) **63**(Suppl):426S–9S.

4   Willett WC, Dietz WH, Colditz GA, Guidelines for healthy weight, *N Engl J Med* (1999) **341**:427–34.

5   Björntorp P, Abdominal obesity and the development of non-insulin-dependent diabetes mellitus, *Diabetes Metab Rev* (1988) **4**:615–22.

6   Chan JM, Stampfer MJ, Ribb EB et al, Obesity, fat distribution and weight gain as risk factors for clinical diabetes in man, *Diabetes Care* (1994) **17**:961–9.

7   Wannamethee SG, Shaper AG, Weight change and duration of overweight and obesity in the incidence of type 2 diabetes, *Diabetes Care* (1999) **22**:1266–72.

8   Sakurai Y, Duration of obesity and risk of non-insulin-dependent diabetes mellitus, *Biomed Pharmacother* (2000) **54**:80–4.

9   Scheen AJ, Aggressive weight reduction treatment in the management of type 2 diabetes, *Diabetes Metab* (1998) **23**:116–23.

10 Scheen AJ, Lefèbvre PJ, Management of the obese diabetic patient, *Diabetes Rev* (1999) **7**:77–93.

11 Scheen AJ, Lefèbvre PJ, Antiobesity

pharmacotherapy in the management of type 2 diabetes, *Diabetes Metab Res Rev* (2000) **16**:114–24.

12 Scheen AJ, Treatment of diabetes in patients with severe obesity, *Biomed Pharmacother* (2000) **54**:74–9.

13 O'Keefe JH, Miles JM, Harris WH et al, Improving the adverse cardiovascular prognosis of type 2 diabetes, *Mayo Clin Proc* (1999) **74**:171–80.

14 Yki-Järvinen H, Role of insulin resistance in the pathogenesis of NIDDM, *Diabetologia* (1995) **38**:1378–88.

15 Scheen AJ, From obesity to diabetes. Why, when and who? *Acta Clin Belg* (2000) **55**:9–15.

16 Zimmet P, Alberti KGMM, Leptin: is it important in diabetes? *Diabetic Med* (1996) **13**:501–3.

17 Taylor SI, Barr V, Reitman M, Does leptin contribute to diabetes caused by obesity? *Science* (1996) **274**:1151–2.

18 Frühbeck G, Salvador J, Relation between leptin and the regulation of glucose metabolism, *Diabetologia* (2000) **43**:3–12.

19 Steppan CM, Bailey ST, Bhat S et al, The hormone resistin links obesity to diabetes. *Nature* (2001) **409**:307–12.

20 Scheen AJ, Castillo MJ, Paquot N, Lefèbvre PJ, How to measure insulin action in vivo, *Diabetes Metab Rev* (1994) **10**:151–88.

21 Scheen AJ, Paquot N, Letiexhe MR et al, Glucose metabolism in obese subjects: lessons from OGTT, IVGTT and clamp studies, *Int J Obesity* (1995) **19**(Suppl 3):S14–S20.

22 Scheen AJ, Lefèbvre PJ, Assessment of insulin resistance in vivo. Application to the study of type 2 diabetes, *Horm Res* (1992) **38**:19–27.

23 Scheen AJ, Paolisso G, Salvatore T, Lefèbvre PJ, Improvement of insulin-induced glucose disposal in obese patients with NIDDM after 1-wk treatment with d-fenfluramine, *Diabetes Care* (1991) **14**:325–32.

24 Reaven GM, Role of insulin resistance in human disease, *Diabetes* (1988) **37**:1595–607.

25 DeFronzo RA, Ferrannini E, Insulin resistance: a multifaceted syndrome responsible for NIDDM, obesity, hypertension, dyslipidemia, and atherosclerotic cardiovascular disease, *Diabetes Care* (1991) **14**:173–94.

26 Haffner SM, D'Agostino R Jr, Mykkänen L et al, Insulin sensitivity in subjects with type 2 diabetes. Relationship to cardiovascular risk factors: the Insulin Resistance Atherosclerosis Study, *Diabetes Care* (1999) **22**:562–8.

27 Henry RR, Type 2 diabetes care: the role of insulin-sensitizing agents and practical implications for cardiovascular disease prevention, *Am J Med* (1998) **105**(Suppl 1A):20S–26S.

28 Després JP, Abdominal obesity as an important component of insulin-resistance syndrome, *Nutrition* (1993) **9**:452–9.

29 Goodpasture BH, Kelley DE, Wing RR et al, Effects of weight loss on regional fat distribution and insulin sensitivity in obesity, *Diabetes* (1999) **48**:839–47.

30 Reaven GM, The fourth Musketeer – from Alexandre Dumas to Claude Bernard, *Diabetologia* (1995) **38**:3–13.

31 Boden G, Role of fatty acids in the pathogenesis of insulin resistance and NIDDM, *Diabetes* (1997) **45**:3–10.

32 Forouhi NG, Jenkinson G, Thomas EL et al, Relation of triglyceride stores in skeletal muscle cells to central obesity and insulin

sensitivity in European and South Asian men, *Diabetologia* (1999) **42**:932–5.

33   Perseghin G, Scifo P, De Cobelli F et al, Intramyocellular triglyceride content is a determinant of in vivo insulin resistance in humans: a ^{1}H-^{13}C nuclear magnetic resonance spectroscopy assessment in offspring of type 2 diabetic parents, *Diabetes* (1999) **48**:1600–6.

34   Hotamisligil GS, Spiegelman BM, Tumor necrosis factor-α: a key component of the obesity–diabetes link, *Diabetes* (1994) **43**:1271–8.

35   Saghizadeh M, Ong JM, Garvey WT et al, The expression of TNFα by human muscle: relationship to insulin resistance, *J Clin Invest* (1996) **97**:1111–16.

36   Ofei F, Hurel S, Newkirk J et al, Effects of an engineered human anti-TNF-α antibody (CDP571) on insulin sensitivity and glycemic control in patients with NIDDM, *Diabetes* (1996) **45**:881–5.

37   Paquot N, Castillo MJ, Lefèbvre PJ, Scheen AJ, No increased insulin sensitivity after a single intravenous administration of a recombinant human tumor necrosis factor receptor: Fc fusion protein in obese insulin-resistant patients, *J Clin Endocrinol Metab* (2000) **85**:1316–19.

38   Baron AD, Hemodynamic actions of insulin, *Am J Physiol* (1994) **30**:E187–202.

39   Wiernsperger N, Vascular defects in the aetiology of peripheral insulin resistance in diabetes. A critical review of hypotheses and facts, *Diabetes Metab Rev* (1994) **10**:287–307.

40   Torlone E, Rambotti AM, Perriello G et al, ACE-inhibition increases hepatic and extrahepatic sensitivity to insulin in patients with type II (non-insulin-dependent) diabetes mellitus and arterial hypertension, *Diabetologia* (1991) **34**:119–25.

41   Donnelly R, Angiotensin-converting enzyme inhibitors and insulin sensitivity: metabolic effects in hypertension, diabetes, and heart failure, *J Cardiovasc Pharmacol* (1992) **20**(Suppl 11):S38–44.

42   Polonsky KS, Sturis J, Bell GI, Non-insulin-dependent diabetes mellitus: a genetically programmed failure of the beta cell to compensate for insulin resistance, *N Engl J Med* (1996) **334**:777–84.

43   Yki-Järvinen H, Glucose toxicity, *Endocr Rev* (1992) **15**:415–31.

44   Unger RH, Lipotoxicity in the pathogenesis of obesity-dependent NIDDM. Genetic and clinical implications, *Diabetes* (1995) **44**:863–70.

45   McGarry, JD, Dobbins RL, Fatty acids, lipotoxicity and insulin secretion, *Diabetologia* (1999) **42**:128–38.

46   Ferrannini E, Insulin resistance vs. insulin deficiency in non-insulin dependent diabetes mellitus: problems and prospects, *Endocr Rev* (1998) **19**:477–90.

47   Turner RC, Cull CA, Frighi V, Holman RR for the UK Prospective Diabetes Study (UKPDS) Group, Glycemic control with diet, sulfonylurea, metformin, or insulin in patients with type 2 diabetes mellitus. Progressive requirement for multiple therapies (UKPDS 49), *JAMA* (1999) **281**:2005–12.

48   Golay A, Felber JP, Evolution from obesity to diabetes, *Diab Metab* (1994) **20**:3–14.

49   Weyer C, Bogardus C, Mott DM, Pratley RE, The natural history of insulin secretory dysfunction and insulin resistance in the pathogenesis of type 2 diabetes mellitus, *J Clin Invest* (1999) **104**:787–94.

50   Leahy JL, Impaired β-cell function with

chronic hyperglycemia: 'overworked β-cell' hypothesis, *Diabetes Rev* (1996) 4:298–319.

51 Weyer C, Hanson K, Bogardus C, Pratley RE, Long-term changes in insulin action and insulin secretion associated with gain, loss, regain and maintenance of body weight, *Diabetologia* (2000) 43:36–46.

52 Scheen AJ, Lefèbvre PJ, Insulin resistance vs. insulin deficiency: which comes first? The old question revisited. In: Di Mario U, Leonetti F, Pugliese G et al, eds, *Diabetes in the New Millennium* (Wiley: New York, 2000) 10–13.

53 Scheen AJ, Luyckx FH, Desaive C, Lefèbvre PJ, Severe/extreme obesity: a medical disease requiring a surgical treatment? *Acta Clin Belg* (1999) 54:154–61.

54 Letiexhe MR, Scheen AJ, Gérard PL et al, Post-gastroplasty recovery of ideal body weight normalizes glucose and insulin metabolism in obese women, *J Clin Endocrinol Metab* (1995) 80:393–9.

55 Luyckx FH, Scheen AJ, Desaive C et al, Effects of gastroplasty on body weight and related biological abnormalities in morbid obesity, *Diab Metab* (1998) 24:355–61.

56 Luyckx FH, Scheen AJ, Desaive C et al, Parallel reversibility of biological markers of the metabolic syndrome and liver steatosis after gastroplasty-induced weight loss in severe obesity (letter), *J Clin Endocrinol Metab* (1999) 84:4293.

57 Brown SA, Upchurch S, Anding R et al, Promoting weight loss in type II diabetes, *Diabetes Care* (1996) 19:613–24.

58 Maggio CA, Pi-Sunyer FX, The prevention and treatment of obesity. Application to type 2 diabetes, *Diabetes Care* (1997) 20:1744–66.

59 Franz MJ, Lifestyle modifications for diabetes management, *Endocrinol Metab Clin North Am* (1997) 26:499–510.

60 American Diabetes Association, Position Statement. Nutrition recommendations and principles for people with diabetes mellitus, *Diabetes Care* (2000) 23(Suppl 1):S43–6.

61 Wing RR, Marcus MD, Epstein LH, Salata R, Type II diabetic subjects lose less weight than their overweight nondiabetic spouses, *Diabetes Care* (1987) 10:563–6.

62 Goldstein DJ, Beneficial health effects of modest weight loss, *Int J Obes* (1992) 16:397–415.

63 Bosello O, Armellini F, Zamboni M, Fitchet M, The benefits of modest weight loss in type II diabetes, *Int J Obesity* (1997) 21(Suppl 1): S10–13.

64 Henry RR, Gumbiner B, Benefits and limitations of very-low-calorie diet therapy in obese NIDDM, *Diabetes Care* (1991) 14:802–23.

65 Scheen AJ, Intérêts et limites de la diète protéique chez le patient obèse diabétique de type 2, *Ann Endocrinol* (1999) 60:103–10.

66 Bray GA, Ryan DH, Drugs used in the treatment of obesity, *Diabetes Rev* (1997) 5:83–103.

67 Scheen AJ, Lefèbvre PJ, Pharmacological treatment of obesity: present status, *Int J Obesity* (1999, 23(Suppl 1):47–53.

68 Carek PJ, Dickerson LM, Current concepts in the pharmacological management of obesity, *Drugs* (1999) 57:883–904.

69 Arnaud O, Nathan C, Antiobesity and lipid-lowering agents with antidiabetic activity. In: Bailey CJ, Flatt PR, eds, *New Antidiabetic Drugs* (Smith-Gordon: Nishimura, 1990) 133–42.

70 Reaven GM, ed, Insulin resistance, hyperinsulinemia and diabetes. Contribution of benfluorex, *Diabetes Metab Rev* (1993) **9**(Suppl 1):S1–72.

71 Giustina A, Rocca I, Romanelli G et al, Effects of benfluorex on glucose tolerance, metabolic control, beta-cell secretion, and peripheral sensitivity to insulin in obese type II diabetic patients on a body weight-maintaining diet, *Curr Ther Res* (1989) **45**:33–42.

72 Cavallo-Perin P, Estivi P, Boine L et al, Benfluorex and blood glucose control in non-insulin-dependent diabetic patients, *J Endocrinol Invest* (1991) **14**:109–13.

73 Bianchi R, Bongers V, Bravenboer B, Erkelens DW, Effects of benfluorex on insulin resistance and lipid metabolism in obese type II diabetic patients, *Diabetes Care* (1993) **16**:557–9.

74 Pontiroli AE, Pacchioni M, Piatti PM et al, Benfluorex in obese noninsulin dependent diabetes mellitus patients poorly controlled by insulin: a double blind study versus placebo, *J Clin Endocrinol Metab* (1996) **81**:3727–32.

75 Leutenegger M, Bauduceau B, Brun JM et al, Added benfluorex in obese insulin-requiring type 2 diabetes, *Diab Metab* (1998) **24**:55–61.

76 Lean MEJ, Sibutramine – a review of clinical efficacy, *Int J Obesity* (1997) **21**(Suppl 1):S30–6.

77 McNeely W, Goa KL, Sibutramine. A review of its contribution in the management of obesity, *Drugs* (1998) **56**:1093–124.

78 Finer N, Bloom SR, Frost GS et al, Sibutramine is effective for weight loss and diabetic control in obesity with type 2 diabetes: a randomised, double-blind, placebo-controlled trial, *Diab Obes Metab* (2000) **2**:1–8.

79 Vargas R, McMahon FG, Jain AK, Effects of sibutramine (S) vs placebo (P) in NIDDM (abstract), *Clin Pharmacol Ther* (1994) **55**:188.

80 Griffiths J, Brynes AE, Frost G et al, Sibutramine in the treatment of overweight non-insulin dependent diabetics (abstract), *Int J Obesity* (1995) **19**(Suppl 2):41.

81 Fujioka K, Weinstein SP, Rowe E et al, Sibutramine induces weight loss and improves glycemic control in obese patients with type 2 diabetes mellitus (abstract), *Diabetologia* (1998) **41**(Suppl 1):A215, 832.

82 Peirce NS, Stubbs TA, MacDonald IA, Tattersall RB, The effect of sibutramine and weight reduction on insulin sensitivity in obese type 2 diabetics (abstract), *Int J Obesity* (1998) **22**(Suppl 3):S272, P669.

83 Rissanen A, for the Finnish Multicentre Group, Sibutramine in the treatment of obese type II diabetics (abstract), *Int J Obesity* (1999) **23**(Suppl 5):S63.

84 Heath MJ, Chong E, Weinstein SP, Seaton TB, Sibutramine enhances weight loss and improves glycemic control and plasma lipid profile in obese patients with type 2 diabetes mellitus (abstract), *Diabetes* (1999) **48**(Suppl 1):A308.

85 Serrano-Rios M, Melchionda N for the Spanish, Italian and Belgian Study Group, Sibutramine is effective for weight loss in obese, sulphonylurea-treated diabetics (abstract), *Int J Obesity* (2000) **24**(Suppl 1):S99.

86 McNulty S, Williams G for the International Study Group, Sibutramine is effective for weight loss in obese, metformin-treated type 2 diabetics (abstract), *Int J Obesity* (2000) **24**(Suppl 1):S100.

87 Rissanen A, Finer N, Fujioka K, Sibutramine-

induced weight loss improves lipid profile in obese type 2 diabetics: results of 3 placebo-controlled, randomized trials (abstract), *Diabetes* (2000, **49**(Suppl 1):A270.

88 Shepherd G, Fitchet M, Kelly F, Sibutramine: a meta-analysis of the change in fasting plasma glucose in patients with a high baseline fasting value (≥5.5 mmol/l) (abstract), *Int J Obesity* (1997) **21**(Suppl 2):S54.

89 Leutenegger M, Hanotin C, Thomas F, Leutenegger E, Sibutramine in the treatment of obese patients presenting a risk of developing diabetes (abstract), *Int J Obesity* (1997) **21**(Suppl 2):S55.

90 Van Gaal LF and the STORM study group, Sibutramine trial of obesity reduction and maintenance. Effects on risk factors (abstract), *Int J Obesity* (1998) **22**(Suppl 3):S272.

91 James WPT, Astrup A, Finer N et al, for the STORM Study Group. Effect of sibutramine on weight maintenance after weight loss: a randomised trial. *Lancet* (2000) **356**:2119–25,

92 Guerciolini R, Mode of action of orlistat, *Int J Obesity* (1997) **21**(Suppl 3):S12–23.

93 McNeely W, Benfield P, Orlistat, *Drugs* (1998) **56**:241–9.

94 Sjöström L, Rissanen A, Andersen T et al, Randomised placebo-controlled trial of orlistat for weight loss and prevention of weight regain in obese patients, *Lancet* (1998) **352**:167–73.

95 Davidson MH, Hauptman J, DiGirolamo M et al, Weight control and risk factor reduction in obese subjects treated for 2 years with orlistat. A randomized controlled trial, *JAMA* (1999) **281**:235–42.

96 Rössner S, Sjöström L, Noack R et al, Weight loss, weight maintenance, and improved cardiovascular risk factors after 2 years

treatment with orlistat for obesity, *Obes Res* (2000) **8**:49–61.

97 Finer N, James WPT, Kopelman PG et al, One-year treatment of obesity: a randomized, double-blind, placebo-controlled, multicentre study of orlistat, a gastrointestinal lipase inhibitor, *Int J Obesity* (2000) **24**:306–13.

98 Heymsfield SB, Segal KR, Hauptman J et al, Effects of weight loss with orlistat on glucose tolerance and progression to type 2 diabetes in obese adults, *Arch Intern Med* (2000) **160**:1321–6.

99 Hollander PA, Elbein SC, Hirsch IB et al, Role of orlistat in the treatment of obese patients with type 2 diabetes. A 1-year randomized double-blind study, *Diabetes Care* (1998) **21**:1288–94.

100 Wilding J, Orlistat-induced weight loss improves insulin resistance in obese patients (abstract), *Diabetologia* (1999) **42**(Suppl 1): A215.

101 Després JP, The impact of orlistat on the multifactorial risk profile of abdominally obese patients (abstract), *Diabetes* (1999) **48**(Suppl 1):A307.

102 Zavoral JH, Treatment with orlistat reduces cardiovascular risk in obese patients, *J Hypertens* (1998) **16**:2013–17.

103 Hollander P, Lucas C, Hauptman J et al, Orlistat reduces body weight and cardiovascular disease risk factors in obese men and women with type 2 diabetes (abstract), *Diabetes* (1999) **48** (Suppl 1), A310.

104 Scheen AJ, Drug treatment of non-insulin-dependent diabetes mellitus in the 1990s: achievements and future developments, *Drugs* (1997) **54**:355–68.

105 DeFronzo RA, Pharmacologic therapy for

type 2 diabetes mellitus, *Ann Intern Med* (1999) **131**:281–303.

106 Scheen AJ, Lefèbvre PJ, Oral antidiabetic agents: a guide to selection, *Drugs* (1998) **55**:225–36.

107 Groop LC, Sulfonylureas and NIDDM, *Diabetes Care* (1992) **15**:737–54.

108 Lebovitz HE, Melander A, Sulfonylureas: basic aspects and clinical uses. In: Alberti KGMM, Zimmet P, DeFronzo RA, Keen H, eds, *International Textbook of Diabetes Mellitus*, 2nd edn (J Wiley: Chichester, 1997) 817–40.

109 United Kingdom Prospective Diabetes Study Group, United Kingdom Prospective Diabetes Study Group 24: A 6-year, randomized, controlled trial comparing sulfonylurea, insulin, and metformin therapy in patients with newly diagnosed type 2 diabetes that could not be controlled with diet therapy, *Ann Intern Med* (1998) **128**:165–75.

110 Cusi K, DeFronzo RA, Metformin: a review of its metabolic effects, *Diabetes Rev* (1998) **6**:89–131.

111 UK Prospective Diabetes Study (UKPDS) Group, Effect of intensive blood-glucose control with metformin on complications in overweight patients with type 2 diabetes (UKPDS 34), *Lancet* (1998) **352**:854–65.

112 Paolisso G, Amato L, Eccellente R et al, Effect of metformin on food intake in obese subjects, *Eur J Clin Invest* (1998) **28**:441–6.

113 Mäkimattila S, Nikkilä K, Yki-Järvinen H, Causes of weight gain during insulin therapy with and without metformin in patients with type II diabetes mellitus, *Diabetologia* (1999) **42**:406–12.

114 The Diabetes Prevention Diabetes Program Research Group, The Diabetes Prevention Program. Design and methods for a clinical trial in the prevention of type 2 diabetes, *Diabetes Care* (1999) **22**:623–34.

115 Balfour JA, McTavish D, Acarbose – an update of its pharmacology and therapeutic use in diabetes mellitus, *Drugs* (1993) **46**:1025–54.

116 Scheen AJ, Clinical efficacy of acarbose in the treatment of diabetes: a critical review of controlled trials, *Diab Metab* (1998) **24**:311–20.

117 Lebovitz HE, α-Glucosidase inhibitors as agents in the treatment of diabetes, *Diabetes Rev* (1998) **6**:132–45.

118 Chiasson JL, Josse RG, Hunt JA et al, The efficacy of acarbose in the treatment of patients with non-insulin-dependent diabetes mellitus: a multicenter controlled clinical trial, *Ann Intern Med* (1994) **121**:928–35.

119 Holman R, Cull AC, Turner RC on behalf of the UKPDS Study Group, A randomized double-blind trial of acarbose in type 2 diabetes shows improved glycemic control over 3 years (UK Prospective Diabetes Study 44), *Diabetes Care* (1999) **22**:960–4.

120 Saltiel AR, Olefsky JM, Thiazolidinediones in the treatment of insulin resistance and type II diabetes, *Diabetes* (1996) **45**:1661–9.

121 Spiegelman BM, PPAR-gamma: adipogenic regulator and thiazolidinedione receptor, *Diabetes* (1998) **47**:507–14.

122 Scheen AJ, Lefèbvre PJ, Troglitazone: antihyperglycemic activity and potential role in the treatment of type 2 diabetes, *Diabetes Care* (1999) **22**:1568–77.

123 Saleh YM, Mudaliar SR, Henry RR, Metabolic and vascular effects of the thiazolidinedione troglitazone, *Diabetes Rev* (1999) **7**:55–76.

124 Shimizu H, Tsuchiya T, Sato N et al, Troglitazone reduces plasma leptin concentrations but increases hunger in NIDDM patients, *Diabetes Care* (1998) **21**:1470–4.

125 Genuth S, Insulin use in NIDDM, *Diabetes Care* (1990) **13**:1240–64.

126 Turner RC, Holman RR, Insulin use in NIDDM. Rationale based on pathophysiology of disease, *Diabetes Care* (1990) **13**:1011–20.

127 Scheen AJ, Insulin therapy in the treatment of NIDDM, *IDF Bulletin* (1996) **41**:16–8.

128 Hayward RA, Manning WG, Kaplan SH et al, Starting insulin therapy in patients with type 2 diabetes. Effectiveness, complications, and resource utilization, *JAMA* (1997) **278**:1663–9.

129 Yki-Järvinen H, Ryysy L, Kauppila M et al, Effects of obesity on the response to insulin therapy in noninsulin-dependent diabetes mellitus, *J Clin Endocrinol Metab* (1997) **82**:4037–43.

130 Scheen AJ, Paquot N, Triches K et al, Traitement ultime du diabète de type 2: insulinothérapie intensive ou chirurgie bariatrique? In: *Journées de Diabétologie de l'Hôtel-Dieu* (Flammarion Médecine-Sciences: Paris, 1998) 81–97.

131 Kerr D, Cavan D, Treating obese patients with poorly controlled diabetes: confessions of an insulin therapist, *Diabetes Metab Res Rev* (1999) **15**:219–25.

132 Scheen AJ, Castillo MJ, Lefèbvre PJ, Combination of oral antidiabetic drugs and insulin in the treatment of non-insulin-dependent diabetes, *Acta Clin Belg* (1993) **48**:259–68.

133 Yki-Järvinen H, Kauppila M, Kujansuu E et al, Comparison of insulin regimens in patients with non-insulin-dependent diabetes mellitus, *N Engl J Med* (1992) **327**:1426–33.

134 Johnson JL, Wolf SL, Kabadi UM, Efficacy of insulin and sulfonylurea combination therapy in type II diabetes. A meta-analysis of the randomized placebo-controlled trials, *Arch Intern Med* (1996) **156**:259–64.

135 Golay A, Guillet-Dauphiné N, Fendel A et al, The insulin-sparing effect of metformin in insulin-treated diabetic patients, *Diabetes Metab Rev* (1995) **11**(Suppl 1):S63–7.

136 Daniel JR, Hagmeyer KO, Metformin and insulin: is there a role for combination therapy? *Ann Pharmacother* (1997) **31**:474–80.

137 Giugliano D, Quatraro A, Consoli G et al, Metformin for obese, insulin-treated diabetic patients: improvements in glycaemic control and reduction of metabolic risk factors, *Eur J Clin Pharmacol* (1993) **44**:107–12.

138 Schwartz S, Raskin P, Fonseca V, Graveline JF for the Troglitazone and Exogenous Insulin Study Group, Effect of troglitazone in insulin-treated patients with type II diabetes mellitus, *N Engl J Med* (1998) **338**:861–6.

139 Coniff RF, Shapiro JA, Seaton TB et al, A double-blind placebo-controlled trial evaluating the safety and efficacy of acarbose for the treatment of patients with insulin-requiring type II diabetes, *Diabetes Care* (1995) **18**:928–32.

140 National Institutes of Health Consensus Development Conference Statement, Gastrointestinal surgery for severe obesity, *Am J Clin Nutr* (1992) **55**:615S–19S.

141 Long SD, O'Brien K, MacDonald KG et al, Weight loss in severely obese subjects prevents

the progression of impaired glucose tolerance to type II diabetes. A longitudinal intervention study, *Diabetes Care* (1993) 17:372–5.

142 Sjöström CD, Lissner L, Wedel H, Sjöström L, Reduction in incidence of diabetes, hypertension and lipid disturbances after intentional weight loss induced by bariatric surgery: the SOS Intervention Study, *Obes Res* (1999) 7:477–84.

143 Pories WJ, MacDonald KG, Flickinger EG et al, Is type II diabetes mellitus (NIDDM) a surgical disease? *Ann Surg* (1992) 215:633–43.

144 Pories WJ, Swanson MS, MacDonald KG et al, Who would have thought it? An operation proves to be the most effective therapy for adult-onset diabetes mellitus, *Ann Surg* (1995) **222**:339–52.

145 Kral JG, Surgical treatment of obesity, In: GA Bray, C Bouchard, WPT James, eds, *Handbook of Obesity* (M Dekker: New York, Basel, Hong Kong, 1998) 977–93.

146 MacDonald KG, Long SD, Swanson MS et al, The gastric bypass operation reduces the progression and mortality on non-insulin-dependent diabetes mellitus, *J Gastrointest Surg* (1997) **1**:213–20.

Obesity and hyperlipidemia

Isabelle Lemieux and Jean-Pierre Després

3

Introduction

It is well established that there is a higher prevalence of chronic metabolic diseases such as hypertension, diabetes and cardiovascular diseases in obese patients than in normal weight individuals.[1–4] However, obesity is heterogeneous in terms of both its etiology and metabolic complications. A French physician from the University of Marseille, Jean Vague, was the first to foresee, through remarkable clinical observations reported in the mid-1940s, that body fat distribution was more important than excess weight per se as a correlate of the complications of obesity.[5] Since this time, these pioneering observations have been supported by hundreds of papers, published mainly over the last two decades. For instance, several prospective studies have shown that a high accumulation of upper body fat is associated with an increased risk of developing type 2 diabetes and coronary heart disease (CHD), and with the mortality related to these complications.[6–11] These prospective studies have all used simple anthropometric measurements, such as the ratio of waist to hip circumferences, to evaluate the distribution of adipose tissue. Metabolic studies have also shown that a high accumulation of abdominal adipose tissue is associated with atherogenic and diabetogenic disturbances such as insulin resistance, hyperinsulinemia, glucose intolerance, dyslipoproteinemias and hypertension.[12–18]

Obesity and metabolic complications

More than 35 years ago, Albrink was the first to re-emphasize Vague's concept when she reported significant associations between trunk fatfolds and fasting triglyceride concentrations which were of higher magnitude than for peripheral skinfolds.[19] Since then, the relationships between indices of body fat distribution and plasma lipoprotein–lipid variables have been extensively documented, mainly with the use of simple anthropometric measurements such as circumferences and skinfolds. With these indices, it has been reported that a high accumulation of abdominal fat is associated with a deterioration in the plasma lipoprotein–lipid profile, including elevated triglyceride[20–22] and apolipoprotein (apo) B levels[23,24] and reduced HDL cholesterol concentrations,[22,25,26] especially in the HDL_2 subfraction.[27–29] Furthermore, no relationships, or very weak relationships, have been reported between plasma cholesterol or LDL cholesterol levels and abdominal fat accumulation.[15,30] However, studies that have directly assessed LDL concentration or

measured the composition, density and size of LDL particles have reported that a high accumulation of adipose tissue in the abdominal region, as crudely assessed by an elevated waist to hip ratio (WHR), was associated with an increased concentration and proportion in the plasma of small, dense, cholesteryl ester-depleted LDL particles. Furthermore, it was found that these substantial quantitative and qualitative changes in LDL could not be appreciated from the conventional LDL cholesterol measurement estimated from precipitation techniques and the Friedewald equation.[28,31,32]

Although the WHR has been the anthropometric variable most frequently used to estimate the proportion of abdominal fat, this measurement does not facilitate the differentiation of subcutaneous fat from visceral adipose tissue. Furthermore, it is important to emphasize that the WHR is an index of the *relative* accumulation of abdominal fat and not of the absolute amount of abdominal adipose tissue. With the development of imaging techniques, such as computed tomography, it has become possible to measure directly, with a high level of accuracy, cross-sectional areas of abdominal subcutaneous and visceral adipose tissue. Studies conducted with this imaging technique revealed significant associations between visceral adipose tissue deposition and metabolic complications.[33–35] Furthermore, it was also found that among obese patients, those with the highest accumulation of visceral adipose tissue were characterized by the most substantial alterations in a cluster of metabolic risk variables.[16,36]

Obesity and dyslipidemia: the importance of visceral obesity

Computed tomography studies have shown that a high accumulation of visceral adipose tissue was associated with an altered plasma lipoprotein–lipid profile in both genders.[15,17,36–40] For instance, we have previously reported that abdominal obesity is associated with increased plasma triglyceride levels and reduced HDL cholesterol concentrations.[24,36] These associations appeared to be independent from the concomitant variation in the level of total body fat.[24,36] To isolate further the independent contribution of visceral adipose tissue from excess fatness, two groups of obese subjects were matched for their percentage of body fat, but were classified on the basis of their low or high levels of visceral adipose tissue and their metabolic profile was then compared to a group of lean controls[24,36] (Figure 3.1). While obese subjects characterized by low levels of visceral adipose tissue had essentially a normal plasma lipoprotein–lipid profile, obese men

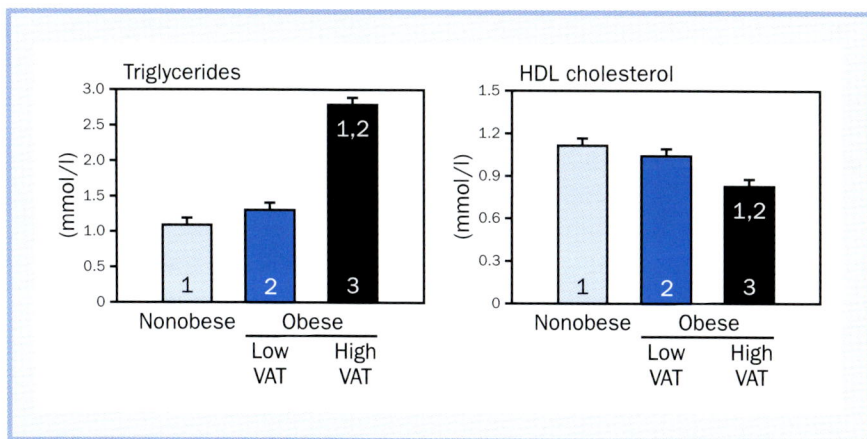

Figure 3.1
Plasma lipoprotein levels in two groups of obese men matched for indices of total body fat, but with either a low or a high accumulation of visceral adipose tissue (VAT) measured by computed tomography. These two subgroups of obese men were compared to a group of nonobese control men. 1: Significantly different from group 1; 2: significantly different from group 2, P < 0.05. (Adapted from Pouliot et al, Diabetes (1992) **41**:826–34.)

with high levels of visceral adipose tissue showed a marked deterioration in their plasma lipoprotein–lipid profile.[24,36] Furthermore, obese patients with a high accumulation of visceral fat showed a marked increase in apo B concentration (25%).[41] Visceral adipose tissue accumulation was also associated with alterations in the size of LDL particles, as viscerally obese men were characterized by an increased proportion of small, dense LDL particles despite an apparent lack of difference in LDL cholesterol levels with lean controls[40] (Figure 3.2). Although there was an association between the small, dense LDL phenotype and the amount of visceral adipose tissue, we have previously reported that visceral obesity was not an independent predictor of an increased proportion of small, dense LDL particles as this phenomenon was largely explained by the hypertriglyceridemic state which was the consequence of the excess accumulation of visceral fat. Indeed, fasting triglyceride concentration was found to be the best predictor of LDL size, whereas LDL cholesterol concentration has no ability to predict variation in LDL particle diameter (Figure 3.3).

Visceral obesity and plasma glucose–insulin homeostasis

In the first study that we conducted on the topic more than a decade ago, we measured body fat distribution by computed tomography and plasma glucose and insulin levels both in the fasting state and after a 75 g oral glucose load in a sample of premenopausal women.[16] We found that the absolute amount of fat located in the abdominal cavity, the so-called visceral adipose tissue, was an important correlate of an impaired glucose tolerance and of elevated insulin concentrations.[16] The level of visceral adipose tissue was the body fat distribution variable which showed the highest association with the area under the curve of the plasma glucose concentrations measured during the oral glucose tolerance test.[16] After control for total adipose tissue mass, the accumulation of visceral adipose tissue remained significantly associated with glucose tolerance.[16] To dissociate further the contribution of obesity versus visceral adipose tissue to disturbances in plasma glucose–insulin homeostasis, obese subjects matched for age and percentage of body fat, but with either low or elevated amounts of visceral adipose tissue, were compared to lean controls (Figure 3.4).[42] Whereas obese men characterized by low levels of visceral fat showed normal glucose tolerance and no difference in plasma insulin concentrations as compared to lean controls, greater glycemic and insulinemic responses were noted among men characterized by elevated levels of visceral adipose tissue.[42]

Similar results emphasizing the importance of visceral adipose tissue as a correlate of an impaired plasma glucose–insulin homeostasis

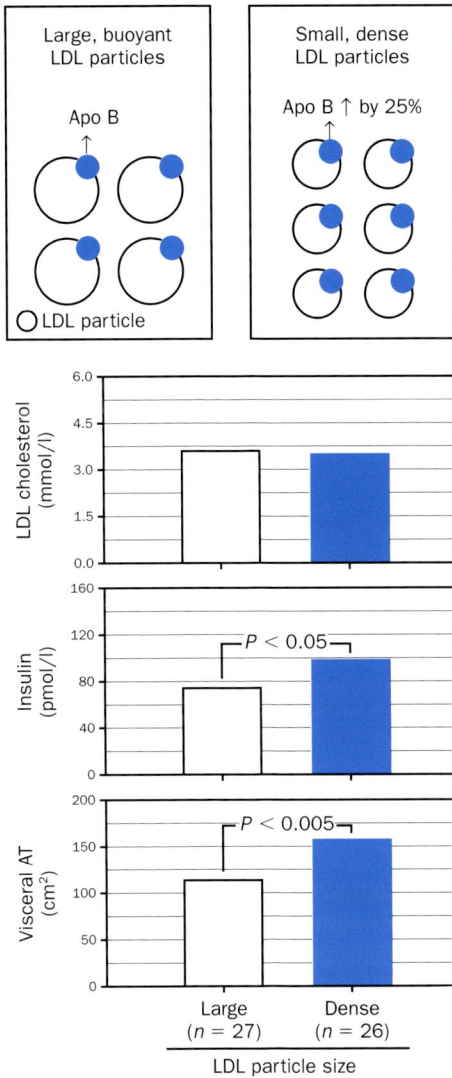

Figure 3.2
LDL peak particle diameter measured by 2–16% polyacrylamide gel electrophoresis and apolipoprotein (Apo) B concentration in two groups of men classified on the basis of body fatness and visceral adipose tissue (AT) accumulation. The two groups of obese men were matched for total body fatness but characterized by either a high or a low accumulation of visceral AT as measured by computed tomography. No difference in LDL cholesterol was found between the two groups (Adapted from Tchernof et al, Diabetes Care (1996) **19:***629–37.)*

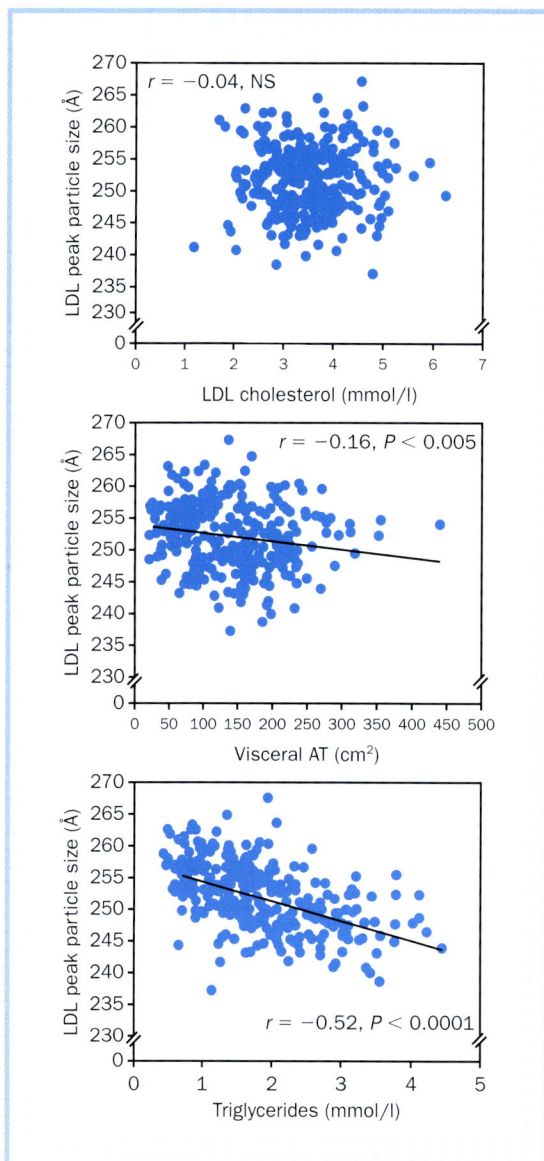

Figure 3.3
Scatter plots of the associations between plasma LDL cholesterol, visceral adipose tissue (AT) accumulation measured by computed tomography, fasting plasma triglycerides and LDL particle size measured by 2–16% polyacrylamide gradient gel electrophoresis in a sample of 299 men.

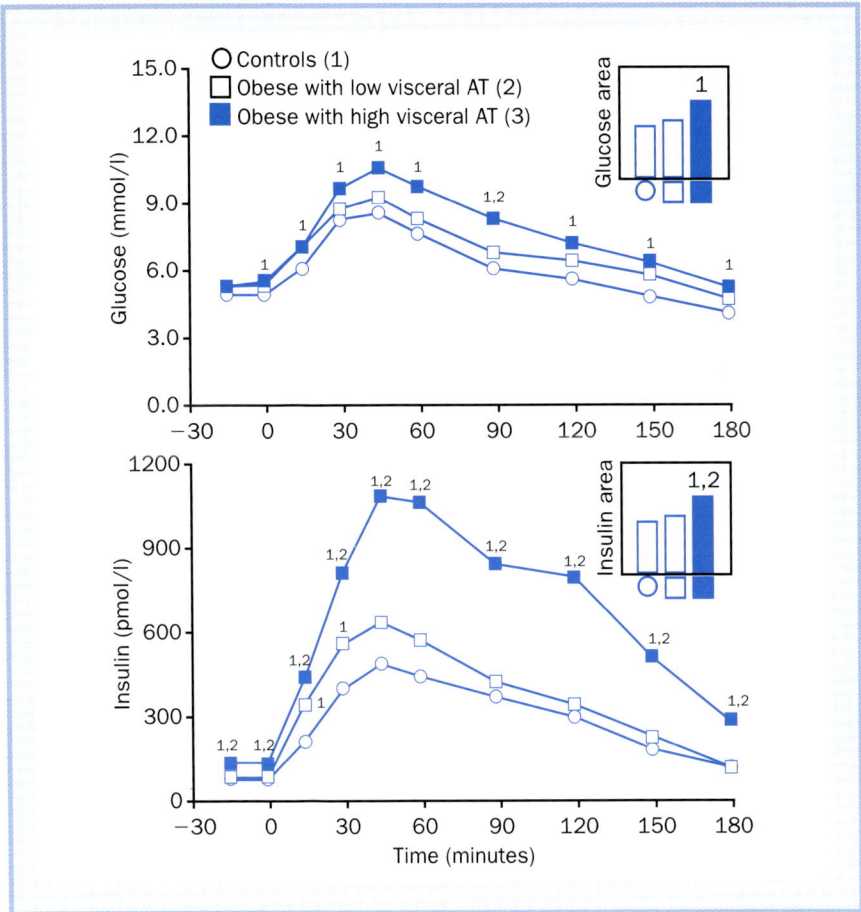

Figure 3.4
*Plasma glucose and insulin levels measured in the fasting state (−15 and 0 min) and after a 75 g oral glucose load in three groups of men. The two groups of obese men were matched for total body fatness, but characterized by either a high or a low accumulation of visceral adipose tissue (AT) measured by computed tomography, and compared to a group of nonobese controls. 1: Significantly different from group 1; 2: significantly different from group 2, P < 0.05. (Adapted from Pouliot et al, Diabetes (1992) **41:**826–34.)*

were obtained in both men and women.[36] Thus among obese subjects, the amount of visceral adipose tissue is predictive of fasting plasma insulin concentrations and of elevated plasma insulin–glucose responses to an oral glucose load, independent of the degree of obesity.[36]

In accordance with these previous results, many studies using computed tomography have provided evidence for an important role of the abdominal visceral fat depot in the etiology of the disturbances in carbohydrate metabolism that are often found in obese patients.[36,38,43–47] In addition, a prospective study has also shown that visceral obesity was associated with an increased risk of developing type 2 diabetes mellitus.[48] Therefore, there is significant evidence suggesting that among obese patients, the most severe disturbances in indices of plasma glucose–insulin homeostasis are observed in patients with a high accumulation of visceral adipose tissue. These alterations are the result of the state of insulin resistance which is found in the viscerally obese patients.

Abdominal obesity as an important component of the insulin resistance syndrome

It therefore appears that abdominal visceral obesity is related to in vivo insulin resistance and to an atherogenic dyslipidemia. In 1988, Reaven was the first to coin the term 'insulin resistance syndrome' to describe a cluster of metabolic abnormalities that included hyperinsulinemia, hypertriglyceridemia, low HDL cholesterol levels as well as elevated blood pressure.[49] To this basic cluster of abnormalities were then added further metabolic alterations which included atherogenic small, dense LDL particles and elevated apo B concentrations as additional elements of this syndrome.[50] Reaven has estimated the prevalence of insulin resistance to reach about 25% of the adult sedentary population, even among nondiabetic subjects.[49] It is important to point out that even in the absence of marked elevations in LDL cholesterol concentrations, this insulin resistant state is associated with an atherogenic dyslipidemic profile which also substantially increases the risk of CHD (Figure 3.5). As visceral adipose tissue accumulation is associated with this cluster of metabolic disturbances leading to an increased risk of type 2 diabetes and CHD, we have proposed that abdominal visceral obesity should be considered as another important component of the insulin resistance syndrome but most importantly, as a central causal factor responsible for these clustering atherogenic abnormalities.[14,50] Although there is limited evidence on visceral obesity as an independent risk factor for CHD it is, however, very likely that the elevated CHD risk noted in viscerally obese individuals is mediated by the large set of clustering abnormalities observed in these patients.

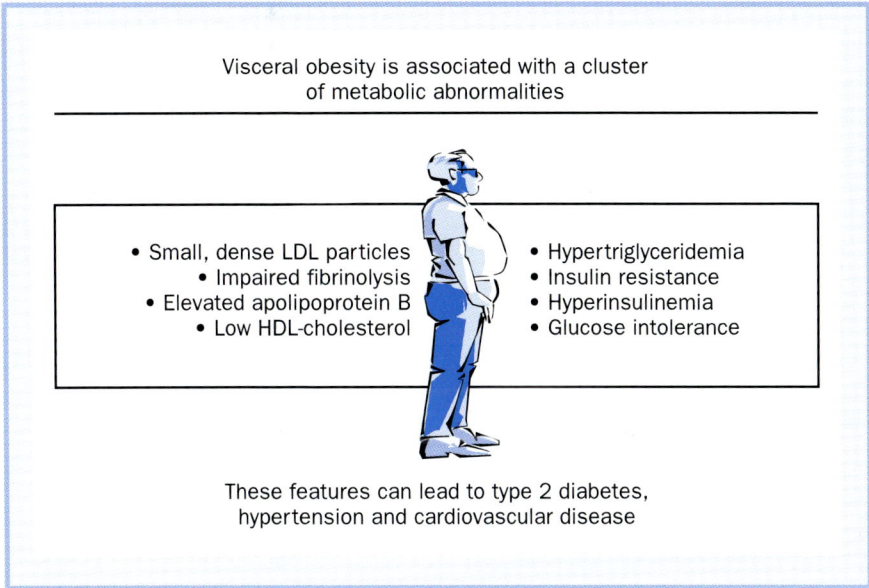

Visceral obesity is associated with a cluster
of metabolic abnormalities

- Small, dense LDL particles
- Impaired fibrinolysis
- Elevated apolipoprotein B
- Low HDL-cholesterol

- Hypertriglyceridemia
- Insulin resistance
- Hyperinsulinemia
- Glucose intolerance

These features can lead to type 2 diabetes,
hypertension and cardiovascular disease

Figure 3.5
*Visceral obesity is associated with the cluster of metabolic abnormalities of the insulin resistance syndrome.
Even in the absence of hyperglycemia and of type 2 diabetes, this cluster substantially increases the risk of
coronary heart disease.*

The dyslipidemic profile of abdominal obesity: implications for CHD risk

Our laboratory has had a long-term interest in the metabolic complications associated with an excessive deposition of visceral adipose tissue.[14,16,27,30,36,40,44,50] Overall, we found visceral abdominal obesity to be associated, even in nondiabetic subjects, with all the features of the insulin resistance syndrome such as hyperinsulinemia, a greater glycemic response to an oral glucose load, elevated triglyceride and apo B concentrations, reduced HDL cholesterol levels, an increased cholesterol/HDL cholesterol ratio and a increased proportion of smaller, cholesteryl-ester depleted LDL particles.[14,16,27,30,36,40,44,50] This cluster of metabolic disturbances is, of course, also found in type 2 diabetic patients who are, most of the time, characterized by insulin resistance and abdominal obesity.

These components of the insulin resistance

syndrome have been shown in the cohort of middle-aged men of the prospective Québec Cardiovascular Study to be associated with a substantial increase in the risk of CHD.[51–53] For instance, we reported that apo B concentration was a strong predictor of the occurrence of CHD events over the 5-year follow-up of the study.[51] We have also documented the CHD risk associated with elevated fasting insulin levels as a crude marker of insulin resistance in nondiabetic men of the Québec Cardiovascular Study.[53] In a case-control prospective analysis, men who developed CHD during the follow-up were matched with men who remained event-free for age, body mass index (BMI), smoking habits and alcohol consumption. We found baseline fasting insulin concentrations to be elevated in men who later developed CHD.[53] Multivariate analyses revealed that hyperinsulinemia was an independent predictor of CHD in these men.[53] Finally, a high proportion of small, dense LDL particles, which is another salient feature of the hypertriglyceridemic–low HDL cholesterol dyslipidemia linked to abdominal obesity and insulin resistance, was also associated with an increased risk of CHD in the Québec Cardiovascular Study.[52]

As insulin, apo B and LDL size were all predictors of CHD risk in the Québec Cardiovascular Study and as these metabolic abnormalities are simultaneously found in viscerally obese men, we then investigated whether our ability to discriminate individuals

at high risk for CHD could be improved by measuring these three nontraditional metabolic risk factors (hyperapoB, hyperinsulinemia and small, dense LDL particles) beyond what can be achieved with the use of traditional lipid risk factors (elevated triglyceride and LDL cholesterol concentrations and reduced HDL cholesterol levels).[54] We found that being simultaneously above the median of the distribution for LDL cholesterol and triglyceride concentrations and below the median of the distribution for HDL cholesterol levels (conventional lipid triad) was associated with a 4.4-fold increase in the risk of CHD over the 5-year follow-up period of the study[54] (Figure 3.6). However, being simultaneously above the median of the distribution for apo B and insulin levels and below the median of LDL peak particle size was associated with more than a 20-fold increased risk of CHD and adjustment for levels of LDL cholesterol, triglycerides and HDL cholesterol failed to significantly alter this elevated relative risk, suggesting that this cluster of new metabolic markers could improve our ability to identify individuals at high risk for CHD.[54]

Assessment of CHD risk in abdominally obese patients: importance of measuring waist and fasting triglycerides

As most general physicians do not have access to insulin, apo B and LDL particle size

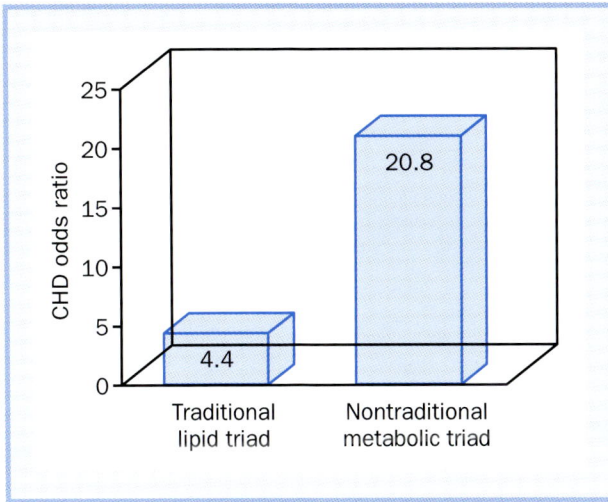

Figure 3.6
The crude odds ratio for developing coronary heart disease (CHD) in a sample of 2103 middle-aged men asymptomatic for CHD and who were followed for incidence of a first CHD event. Over a 5-year follow-up, the CHD odds ratio was increased by 20.8-fold among men who had all three traditional nontraditional risk factors simultaneously (nontraditional metabolic triad: elevated apolipoprotein B and insulin levels and small, dense LDL particles) compared with those who were characterized by all the three traditional risk factors (lipid triad: elevated triglyceride and LDL cholesterol levels and reduced HDL cholesterol concentrations) in whom the odds ratio was 4.4. (Adapted from Lamarche et al.[54])

measurements, we were interested in developing a simple algorithm which could be used in daily clinical practice to identify at low cost, asymptomatic but high-risk individuals, likely to be carriers of this atherogenic metabolic triad.[55]

The working model that we have used to identify carriers of the nontraditional atherogenic metabolic triad included waist girth (which was considered as a proxi variable for insulin and apo B levels) and fasting triglyceride concentration (which was used to screen for the presence of small, dense LDL particles) (Figure 3.7). Since we had

previously suggested that waist girth could be used as a crude index of abdominal visceral adipose tissue accumulation,[56] we felt that a simple anthropometric variable such as the waist circumference could improve the assessment of cardiovascular risk linked to abdominal obesity. In this regard, we have reported that apo B and fasting insulin levels were very sensitive to an increase in waist circumference, resulting from an accumulation of abdominal visceral fat.[55] Accordingly, we found that men between 40 and 65 years of age with an elevated waist circumference ($\geq$90 cm) were characterized

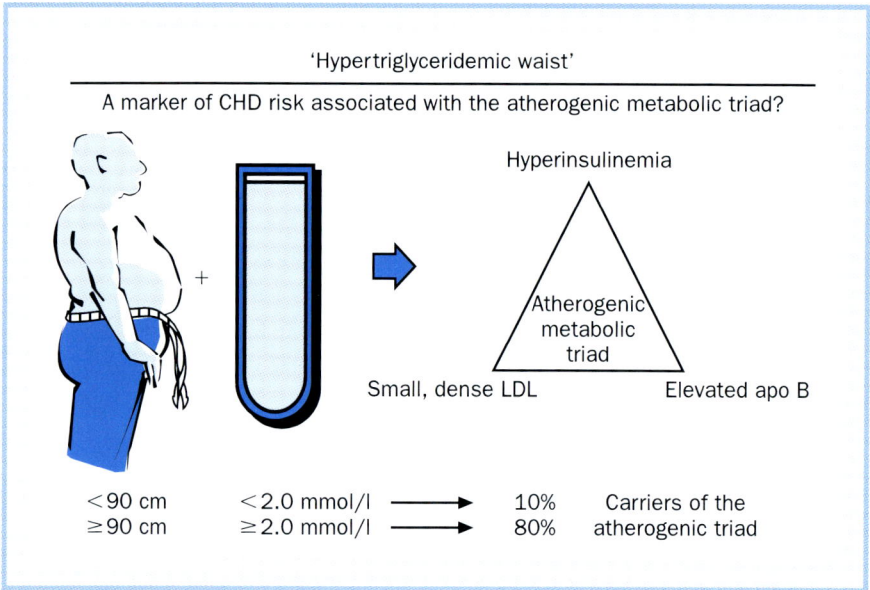

'Hypertriglyceridemic waist'

A marker of CHD risk associated with the atherogenic metabolic triad?

Hyperinsulinemia

Atherogenic metabolic triad

Small, dense LDL   Elevated apo B

| <90 cm | <2.0 mmol/l | → | 10% | Carriers of the |
| ≥90 cm | ≥2.0 mmol/l | → | 80% | atherogenic triad |

Figure 3.7
*Prevalence of carriers of the atherogenic metabolic triad among middle-aged men classified on the basis of waist circumference and fasting triglyceride levels. Apo B: apolipoprotein B. (Adapted from Lemieux et al, Circulation **102**:179–84.)*

by both fasting hyperinsulinemia and increased apo B levels. As fasting triglyceride concentration had been previously reported to be the best predictor of LDL diameter,[40,57,58] we used this variable as a predictor of LDL size and found that men with moderate hypertriglyceridemia (≥2.0 mmol/l) were characterized by a high likelihood of having small, dense LDL particles.

We therefore proposed that the 'hypertriglyceridemic waist' concept may be useful to screen for the presence of the new metabolic triad of atherogenic risk factors. After having divided our cohort of men according to triglyceride levels (<2.0 mmol/l; ≥2.0 mmol/l) and waist girth (<90 cm; 90–100 cm; ≥100 cm), we found that in the absence of elevated triglyceride levels, only 12% and 53% of men with a moderate or a high waist girth were characterized by the atherogenic triad.[55] However, a high proportion of men (more than 80%) with

simultaneous elevations in waist girth
($\geq$90 cm) and triglyceride concentrations
($\geq$2.0 mmol/l) were characterized by the new
triad of metabolic risk factors (Figure 3.7).
Irrespective of the marked alterations in the
unconventional risk variables, it is also
important to point out that these
abdominally-hypertriglyceridemic men were
also characterized by substantial elevations in
the cholesterol/HDL cholesterol ratio (a well
accepted predictor of CHD risk).[59,60] When
we validated this algorithm on another sample
of male patients who underwent an
angiographic evaluation, we found that the
relative likelihood of being affected by
coronary artery disease was only significantly
increased (by 3.6-fold) in the subgroup of
male patients who had both an increased waist
girth and elevated triglyceride
concentrations.[55]

There is also additional evidence
supporting the notion that waist
circumference and triglyceride concentrations
could be used as effective screening tools.
Recent analyses from the Québec Health
Survey revealed that about 50% of men are
characterized by triglyceride levels below
2.0 mmol/l and by a waist girth below
90 cm.[61] However, almost 20% of Québecers
have simultaneous elevations in waist
circumference and triglyceride levels.[61] In
women, 76% presented a waist girth below
90 cm and were characterized by low levels of
triglycerides, whereas only 5% were

characterized by simultaneous elevations in
waist girth and triglyceride concentrations.[61]
In this population-based study of men living
in the province of Québec, we also quantified
the prevalence of an elevated cholesterol/HDL
cholesterol ratio (as defined by a
cholesterol/HDL cholesterol ratio $\geq$6) among
men classified on the basis of waist girth and
triglyceride concentrations.[61] Whereas only
3% of men with low waist girth and low
triglyceride concentrations had a
cholesterol/HDL cholesterol ratio above 6,
almost 50% of men with the
'hypertriglyceridemic waist' were characterized
by a cholesterol/HDL cholesterol ratio ($\geq$6).[61]
Finally, when the subjects' characteristics were
examined across waist girth and triglyceride
groups, it was interesting to note that marked
differences were observed in the
cholesterol/HDL cholesterol ratio in the
absence of any difference in BMI and WHR.[61]
Thus, substantial variation in the
cholesterol/HDL cholesterol ratio was noted
as a function of combined waist and
triglyceride values. For instance, abdominally
obese men with triglyceride levels above
2.0 mmol/l had a cholesterol/HDL cholesterol
ratio of about 1.5 units greater than men with
triglyceride concentrations below 2.0 mmol/l
and with waist girth below 90 cm.[61] Thus, the
combined interpretation of waist
circumference and fasting triglyceride levels
may be superior to the WHR and BMI as
screening tools to identify abdominally obese

men with the atherogenic dyslipidemia of insulin resistance.

The atherogenic dyslipidemia of visceral obesity: implications for prevention and treatment

As the insulin resistance syndrome is a highly prevalent condition with considerable public health implications, there is a need to develop simple and inexpensive screening markers for the identification of individuals at increased risk of developing type 2 diabetes and CHD before the occurrence of the disease. However, as the majority of abdominally obese men at high risk for CHD may never develop type 2 diabetes, it is also of paramount importance to use early markers of the insulin resistance syndrome in order to implement primary prevention strategies focusing on high-risk, abdominally obese patients. On that basis, it has been suggested that fasting hyperinsulinemia could be the simplest and best marker of early insulin resistance in nondiabetic and euglycemic individuals.[62,63] However, measuring fasting insulin concentration is not a routine procedure in most clinical biochemistry laboratories as the assay is not standardized. Meanwhile, a high proportion of nondiabetic individuals with abdominal obesity, who have never smoked and who may never be affected by hypercholesterolemia and hypertension, are

characterized by a cluster of metabolic complications substantially increasing the risk of CHD and type 2 diabetes.

Therefore, assessment of traditional risk factors including the BMI may not be sufficient to evaluate the CHD risk of obese patients properly. Furthermore, one needs to go far beyond cholesterol and LDL cholesterol measurements to assess adequately the atherogenic dyslipidemic state in high-risk obese patients with an excess accumulation of visceral adipose tissue as most of these patients have cholesterol and LDL cholesterol which are either in the 'normal range' or only marginally elevated. It is now increasingly recognized that the atherogenic dyslipidemia of the abdominally obese patient with insulin resistance includes hypertriglyceridemia, low HDL cholesterol levels as well as an increased proportion of small, dense LDL particles accompanied by an increased concentration of atherogenic apo B-containing lipoproteins. Therefore, the clinician will have to pay attention to these metabolic markers of risk and aim beyond LDL cholesterol lowering as a therapeutic target.

As it has been suggested that a moderate weight loss of about 10% could lead to a selective mobilization of visceral fat of about 25–30% in abdominally obese patients (Figure 3.8), it has been suggested that monitoring changes in waist circumference over time may improve the physician's ability to assess the efficacy of treatment (diet,

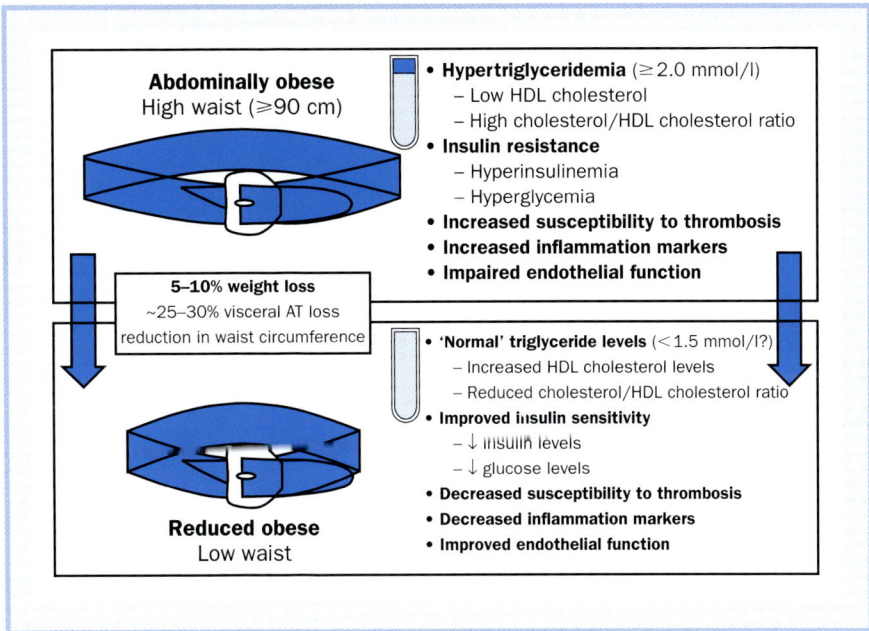

Figure 3.8
Simple markers of the athero-thrombotic inflammatory profile increasing coronary heart disease risk in the abdominally obese patient. Under this theoretical model, moderate weight loss associated with a preferential mobilization of visceral adipose tissue (AT) could significantly reduce the risk of an acute coronary syndrome in these patients. Randomized weight loss trial in abdominally obese patients will have to be conducted to test this model.

physical activity and, if required, pharmacotherapy) aimed at the management of the dyslipidemia and of other CHD risk factors in the obese patient.

In conclusion, in addition to the legitimate pharmacotherapy of hyperglycemia, hypertension or of the dyslipidemia, we would like to propose, from the clustering atherogenic, prothrombotic and inflammatory abnormalities found in abdominally obese patients, that these high-risk individuals will not be properly managed for CHD risk until abdominal obesity (waist girth) is identified as another important therapeutic target. It is therefore proposed that 'waist reduction' should be recognized as an important therapeutic objective for the management of high-risk, dyslipidemic, abdominally obese patients.

Acknowledgments

Studies conducted by the authors discussed in this chapter have benefited from the support of the Canadian Institutes of Health Research (MT-14014 and MGC-15187), the Canadian Diabetes Association and the Heart and Stroke Foundation of Canada. Isabelle Lemieux is the recipient of a research studentship from the Heart and Stroke Foundation of Canada whereas Jean-Pierre Després is chair professor of nutrition, lipidology and prevention of cardiovascular disease supported by Provigo and Pfizer.

References

1 Sims EAH, Berchtold P, Obesity and hypertension: mechanisms and implications for management, *JAMA* (1982) **247**:49–52.

2 Bray GA, Complications of obesity, *Ann Intern Med* (1985) **103**:1052–62.

3 Garrison RJ, Kannel WB, Stokes JD, Castelli WP, Incidence and precursors of hypertension in young adults: the Framingham Offspring Study, *Prev Med* (1987) **16**(2):235–51.

4 Kissebah AH, Peiris AN, Biology of regional body fat distribution: relationship to non-insulin-dependent diabetes mellitus, *Diabetes Metab Rev* (1989) **5**:83–109.

5 Vague J, Sexual differentiation, a factor affecting the forms of obesity, *Presse Méd* (1947) **30**:339–40.

6 Ohlson LO, Larsson B, Svardsudd K et al, The influence of body fat distribution on the incidence of diabetes mellitus. 13.5 years of follow-up of the participants in the study of men born in 1913, *Diabetes* (1985) **34**(10):1055–8.

7 Haffner SM, Stern MP, Mitchell BD, Hazuda HP, Patterson JK, Incidence of type II diabetes in Mexican Americans predicted by fasting insulin and glucose levels, obesity, and body-fat distribution, *Diabetes* (1990) **39**(3):283–8.

8 Lapidus L, Bengtsson C, Larsson B, Pennert K, Rybo E, Sjöström L, Distribution of adipose tissue and risk of cardiovascular disease and death: a 12 year follow up of participants in the population study of women in Gotenburg, Sweden, *Br J Nutr* (1984) **289**:1261–3.

9 Larsson B, Svardsudd K, Welin L, Wilhelmsen L, Björntorp P, Tibblin G, Abdominal adipose tissue distribution, obesity, and risk of cardiovascular disease and death: 13 year follow-up of participants in the study of men born in 1913, *Br Med J* (1984) **288**:1401–4.

10 Ducimetiere P, Richard J, Cambien F, The pattern of subcutaneous fat distribution in middle-aged men and the risk of coronary heart disease: the Paris Prospective Study, *Int J Obes* (1986) **10**(3):229–40.

11 Donahue RP, Abbott RD, Bloom E, Reed DM, Yano K, Central obesity and coronary heart disease in men, *Lancet* (1987) **i**(8537):821–4.

12 Kissebah AH, Freedman DS, Peiris AN, Health risk of obesity, *Med Clin North Am* (1989) **1989**:111–38.

13 Björntorp P, Abdominal obesity and the development of non-insulin dependent diabetes mellitus, *Diabetes Metab Rev* (1988) **4**:615–22.

14 Després JP, Visceral obesity: a component of the insulin resistance-dyslipidemic syndrome, *Can J Cardiol* (1994) **10**:17B–22B.

15 Després JP, Obesity and lipoprotein metabolism: relevance of body fat distribution, *Curr Opin Lipidol* (1991) **2**:5–15.

16 Després JP, Nadeau A, Tremblay A et al, Role of deep abdominal fat in the association between regional adipose tissue distribution and glucose tolerance in obese women, *Diabetes* (1989) **38**:304–9.

17 Després JP, Lipoprotein metabolism in visceral obesity, *Int J Obes* (1991) **15**(Suppl 2):45–52.

18 Kissebah AH, Krakower GR, Regional adiposity and morbidity, *Physiol Rev* (1994) **74**(4):761–811.

19 Albrink MJ, Meigs JW, The relationship between serum triglycerides and skinfold thickness in obese subjects, *Ann NY Acad Sci* (1965) **131**(1):673–83.

20 Kissebah AH, Vydelingum N, Murray R et al, Relation of body fat distribution to metabolic complications of obesity, *J Clin Endocrinol Metab* (1982) **54**(2):254–60.

21 Krotkiewski M, Björntorp P, Sjöström L, Smith U, Impact of obesity on metabolism in men and women. Importance of regional adipose tissue distribution, *J Clin Invest* (1983) **72**:1150–62.

22 Després JP, Allard C, Tremblay A, Talbot J, Bouchard C, Evidence for a regional component of body fatness in the association with serum lipids in men and women, *Metabolism* (1985) **34**:967–73.

23 Galanis DJ, McGarvey ST, Sobal J, Bausserman L, Levinson PD, Relations of body fat and fat distribution to the serum lipid, apolipoprotein and insulin concentrations of Samoan men and women, *Int J Obes Relat Metab Disord* (1995) **19**(10):731–8.

24 Després JP, Dyslipidaemia and obesity, *Baillieres Clin Endocrinol Metab* (1994) **8**(3):629–60.

25 Kissebah AH, Evans DJ, Peiris A, Wilson CR, Endocrine characteristics in regional obesities: role of sex steroids. In: Vague J, Björntorp P, Guy-Grand B, Rebuffe-Scrive M, Vague P, eds, *Metabolic Complications of Human Obesities* (Elsevier: Amsterdam, 1985) 115–30.

26 Anderson AJ, Sobocinski KA, Freedman DS, Barboriak JJ, Rimm AA, Gruchow HW, Body fat distribution, plasma lipids and lipoproteins, *Arterioscler Thromb Vasc Biol* (1988) **8**:88–94.

27 Després JP, Moorjani S, Ferland M et al, Adipose tissue distribution and plasma lipoprotein levels in obese women. Importance of intra-abdominal fat, *Arteriosclerosis* (1989) **9**(2):203–10.

28 Terry RB, Wood PD, Haskell WL, Stefanick ML, Krauss RM, Regional adiposity patterns in relation to lipids, lipoprotein cholesterol, and lipoprotein subfraction mass in men, *J Clin Endocrinol Metab* (1989) **68**(1):191–9.

29 Ostlund RE Jr, Staten M, Kohrt WM, Schultz J, Malley M, The ratio of waist-to-hip circumference, plasma insulin level, and glucose intolerance as independent predictors of the HDL2 cholesterol level in older adults, *N Engl J Med* (1990) **322**(4):229–34.

30 Després JP, Moorjani S, Lupien PJ, Tremblay A, Nadeau A, Bouchard C, Regional distribution of body fat, plasma lipoproteins, and cardiovascular disease, *Arteriosclerosis* (1990) **10**(4):497–511.

31 Peeples LH, Carpenter JW, Israel RG, Barakat HA, Alterations in low-density lipoproteins in subjects with abdominal adiposity, *Metabolism* (1989) **38**(10):1029–36.

32 Després JP, Abdominal obesity as important component of insulin-resistance syndrome, *Nutrition* (1993) **9**(5):452–9.

33 Sjöström L, Kvist H, Cederblad A, Tylen U, Determination of total adipose tissue and body fat in women by computed tomography, 40K, and tritium, *Am J Physiol* (1986) **250**:E736–45.

34 Ferland M, Després JP, Tremblay A et al, Assessment of adipose tissue distribution by computed axial tomography in obese women: association with body density and anthropometric measurements, *Br J Nutr* (1989) **61**(2):139–48.

35 Després JP, Prud'homme D, Pouliot MC, Tremblay A, Bouchard C, Estimation of deep abdominal fat accumulation from simple anthropometric measurements in men, *Am J Clin Nutr* (1991) **54**:471–7.

36 Pouliot MC, Després JP, Nadeau A et al, Visceral obesity in men. Associations with glucose tolerance, plasma insulin, and lipoprotein levels, *Diabetes* (1992) **41**(7):826–34.

37 Peiris AN, Sothmann MS, Hoffmann RG et al, Adiposity, fat distribution, and cardiovascular risk, *Ann Intern Med* (1989) **110**(11):867–72.

38 Fujioka S, Matsuzawa Y, Tokunaga K, Tarui S, Contribution of intra-abdominal fat accumulation to the impairment of glucose and lipid metabolism in human obesity, *Metabolism* (1987) **36**(1):54–9.

39 Lemieux S, Després JP, Moorjani S et al, Are gender differences in cardiovascular disease risk factors explained by the level of visceral adipose tissue?, *Diabetologia* (1994) **37**:757–64.

40 Tchernof A, Lamarche B, Prud'homme D et al, The dense LDL phenotype. Association with plasma lipoprotein levels, visceral obesity, and hyperinsulinemia in men, *Diabetes Care* (1996) **19**(6):629–37.

41 Lemieux S, Després JP, Metabolic complications of visceral obesity: contribution to the aetiology of type 2 diabetes and implications for prevention and treatment, *Diabet Metab* (1994) **20**(4):375–93.

42 Després JP, Visceral obesity, insulin resistance, and related dyslipoproteinemias. In: Diabetes

1991: Proceedings of the 14th International Diabetes Federation Congress, Washington, DC, 23–28 June 1991. Rifkin H, Colwell JA, Taylor SI, eds (Elsevier: Amsterdam, 1991) 95–9.

43 Sparrow D, Borkan GA, Gerzof SG, Wisniewski C, Silbert CK, Relationship of fat distribution to glucose tolerance. Results of computed tomography in male participants of the Normative Aging Study, *Diabetes* (1986) **35**(4):411–5.

44 Després JP, Ferland M, Moorjani S, Nadeau A, Tremblay A, Lupien PJ, Role of hepatic-triglyceride lipase activity in the association between intra-abdominal fat and plasma HDL cholesterol in obese women, *Arterioscler Thromb Vasc Biol* (1989) **9**:485–92.

45 Peiris AN, Sothmann MS, Hennes MI et al, Relative contribution of obesity and body fat distribution to alterations in glucose insulin homeostasis: predictive values of selected indices in premenopausal women, *Am J Clin Nutr* (1989) **49**(5):758–64.

46 Seidell JC, Björntorp P, Ströström L, Kvist H, Sannerstedt R, Visceral fat accumulation in men is positively associated with insulin, glucose, and C-peptide levels, but negatively with testosterone levels, *Metabolism* (1990) **39**(9):897–901.

47 Park KS, Rhee BD, Lee KU et al, Intra-abdominal fat is associated with decreased insulin sensitivity in healthy young men, *Metabolism* (1991) **40**(6):600–3.

48 Bergstrom RW, Newell-Morris LL, Leonetti DL, Shuman WP, Wahl PW, Fujimoto WY, Association of elevated fasting C-peptide level and increased intra-abdominal fat distribution with development of NIDDM in Japanese-American men, *Diabetes* (1990) **39**(1): 104–11.

49 Reaven GM, Banting lecture 1988. Role of insulin resistance in human disease, *Diabetes* (1988) **37**(12):1595–607.

50 Després JP, Marette A, Relation of components of insulin resistance syndrome to coronary disease risk, *Curr Opin Lipidol* (1994) **5**(4):274–89.

51 Lamarche B, Moorjani S, Lupien P-J et al, Apolipoprotein A-I and B levels and the risk of ischemic heart disease during a five-year follow-up of men in the Québec cardiovascular study, *Circulation* (1996) **94**:273–8.

52 Lamarche B, Tchernof A, Moorjani S et al, Small, dense low-density lipoprotein particles as a predictor of the risk of ischemic heart disease in men. Prospective results from the Québec Cardiovascular Study, *Circulation* (1997) **95**:69–75.

53 Després JP, Lamarche B, Mauriège P et al, Hyperinsulinemia as an independent risk factor for ischemic heart disease, *N Engl J Med* (1996) **334**:952–7.

54 Lamarche B, Tchernof A, Mauriège P et al, Fasting insulin and apolipoprotein B levels and low-density lipoprotein particle size as risk factors for ischemic heart disease, *JAMA* (1998) **279**:1955–61.

55 Lemieux I, Pascot A, Couillard C et al, Hypertriglyceridemic waist. A marker of the atherogenic metabolic triad (hyperinsulinemia, hyperapolipoprotein B, small, dense LDL) in men? *Circulation* (2000) **102**:179–84.

56 Pouliot MC, Després JP, Lemieux S et al, Waist circumference and abdominal sagittal diameter: best simple anthropometric indexes of abdominal visceral adipose tissue accumulation and related cardiovascular risk in men and women, *Am J Cardiol* (1994) **73**(7):460–8.

57 Lemieux I, Pascot A, Tchernof A et al, Visceral adipose tissue and low-density lipoprotein particle size in middle-aged versus young men, *Metabolism* (1999) **48**(10):1322–7.

58 McNamara JR, Jenner JL, Li Z, Wilson PW, Schaefer EJ, Change in LDL particle size is associated with change in plasma triglyceride concentration, *Arterioscler Thromb Vasc Biol* (1992) **12**(11):1284–90.

59 Manninen V, Tenkanen L, Koshinen P et al, Joint effects of serum triglyceride and LDL cholesterol and HDL cholesterol concentrations on coronary heart disease risk in the Helsinki Heart Study: implications for treatment, *Circulation* (1992) **85**:37–45.

60 Stampfer MJ, Sacks FM, Salvini S, Willett WC, Hennekens CH, A prospective study of cholesterol, apolipoproteins, and the risk of myocardial infarction, *N Engl J Med* (1991) **325**:373–81.

61 Lemieux I, Alméras N, Mauriège P et al, Waist circumference and triglyceride levels as screening tools for the evaluation of IHD risk in men, *Obes Res* (1999) 7:60S.

62 Ferrannini E, Haffner SM, Mitchell BD, Stern MP, Hyperinsulinaemia: the key feature of a cardiovascular and metabolic syndrome, *Diabetologia* (1991) **34**(6):416–22.

63 Laakso M, How good a marker is insulin level for insulin resistance? *Am J Epidemiol* (1993) **137**:959–65.

Obesity and cardiovascular disease and hypertension

Simon W Coppack

4

Cardiovascular disease as a complication of obesity, the inter-relationships of co-morbidities

As will be clear from other chapters of this book, many of the co-morbidities of obesity are inter-related. This is especially true of cardiovascular disease which usually does not occur as an isolated problem but which is found in subjects already suffering from a range of obesity co-morbidities.[1,2] The management of the heart problems of obesity are then complicated by having to consider treatment (a) for the obesity itself, (b) for any other co-morbidities (such as hypertension) that promote cardiovascular problems and (c) for the cardiac problems per se. Similar complexity affects any discussion of the relationship between obesity and cardiovascular disease.

The co-morbidities associated with obesity are shown in Table 4.1. Of these conditions, some such as arthritis and psychological problems are more likely to cause distress than be a direct cause of mortality. Other co-morbidities such as diabetes and nocturnal hypoventilation cause morbidity directly and also indirectly contribute to mortality (Chapters 2 and 6). These conditions usually promote mortality by acting as risk factors for cardiovascular disease. The two biggest 'direct' causes of death in obese patients are cancer and cardiovascular disease. Several co-morbidities, in particular diabetes and hypertension, cause premature death mainly through cardiovascular disease.

As indicated in Table 4.1, the group of obesity complications that principally cause 'morbidity rather than mortality' also contains some factors that epidemiologists would recognize as being strongly related to cardiovascular disease. Thus depression and mental health problems are epidemiologically linked to cardiovascular mortality in the general population. The same could be said of social disadvantage and low levels of physical fitness.[3] Such interactions make it difficult to apportion the risk of cardiovascular disease to specific risk factors (Figure 4.1). It has been shown, for example by the Framingham study,[4,5] that obesity is an independent risk factor for cardiovascular disease after statistical allowance is made for the 'classic' cardiovascular risk factors of smoking, lipids, diabetes and hypertension. However, it is not known whether this 'independent' effect relationship between obesity and cardiovascular disease is accounted for by low physical fitness, nocturnal hypoventilation,

Table 4.1
Major co-morbidities of obesity.

Co-morbidities principally causing morbidity rather than mortality	*Osteoarthrosis* *Gall stones* *Bladder dysfunction* *Psychological problems including depression, agoraphobia, etc* *Low social status, unemployment and social disadvantage* *Low levels of physical fitness*
Co-morbidities indirectly causing mortality, mostly via cardiovascular disease	*Obstructive sleep apnoea and other nocturnal hypoventilation* *Diabetes* *Dyslipidaemia (hypertriglyceridaemia, low HDL cholesterol, small, dense LDL)* *Hypertension* *Thromboembolic disease*
Co-morbidities directly causing mortality	*Cardiovascular disease including cardiomyopathies,* *Obesity-related cancers such as colonic, uterine, ovarian, gallbladder*

and so forth. The question of whether obesity per se causes cardiovascular disease is, however, somewhat academic. There is no doubt that obesity causes co-morbities and it is somewhat perverse to ignore or 'correct for' these co-morbidities when examining the relationship between obesity and cardiovascular disease.

Epidemiology

Obesity is a major cause of increased cardiovascular disease in the general population.[4] Given that obesity is also the major cause of diabetes and other co-morbities, it has been estimated that obesity (with its co-morbidities) has a total impact on cardiovascular disease in the general population approximately equal to that of smoking and perhaps exceeding that of LDL cholesterol.[6] In terms of current secular trends, cardiovascular disease is declining as a result of reduced smoking, but the decline is offset by increasing obesity.[7]

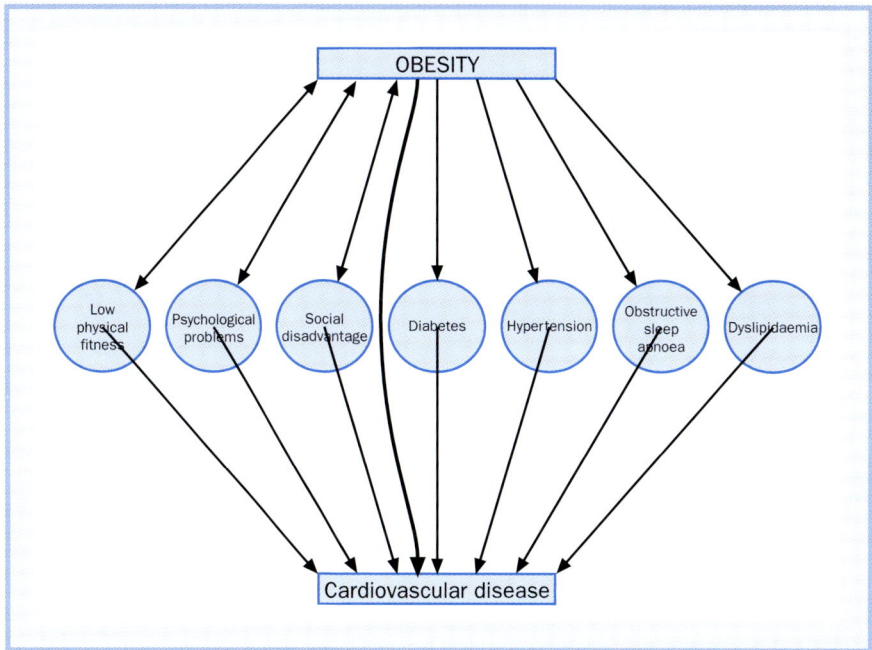

Figure 4.1
Scheme outlining relationships between obesity and cardiovascular disease. Arrows indicate the presumptive causalities of the relationships.

Although there is little doubt that an increase in body mass index (BMI) and percentage ideal body weight (%IBW) are powerful univariate predictors of morbidity, some workers suggest that visceral obesity represents a variant that is more closely related to excess morbidity (see Chapter 3). As discussed in Chapter 1, visceral obesity is usually measured by waist circumference or the waist to hip ratio. One interpretation of the link between morbidity and high waist to hip ratio is that visceral fat has especially 'bad' metabolic actions. Others point to data showing that general adiposity is as dangerous as accumulation in any single region. This second school of thought points out that a high waist to hip ratio is strongly linked to low physical activity,

to recent weight gain and to high alcohol intake.[8] Studies correcting for these factors will be required before the suggestion can be accepted that visceral fat per se has some adverse metabolic effect. This is not to suggest that a large waist circumference is not important: it may be important as an index of physical inactivity.

The relationship between body weight and premature mortality is also complicated by cigarette smoking.[6] Smoking is associated with reduced obesity. Thus if smokers are included in the data the BMI versus mortality relationship is relatively diluted. If only nonsmokers are considered, then there is a clear increased mortality in obese subjects. These relationships are indicated in Figure 4.2 which shows

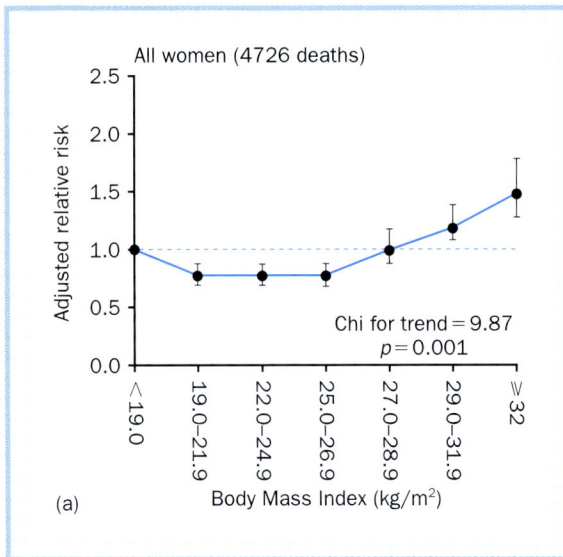

(a)

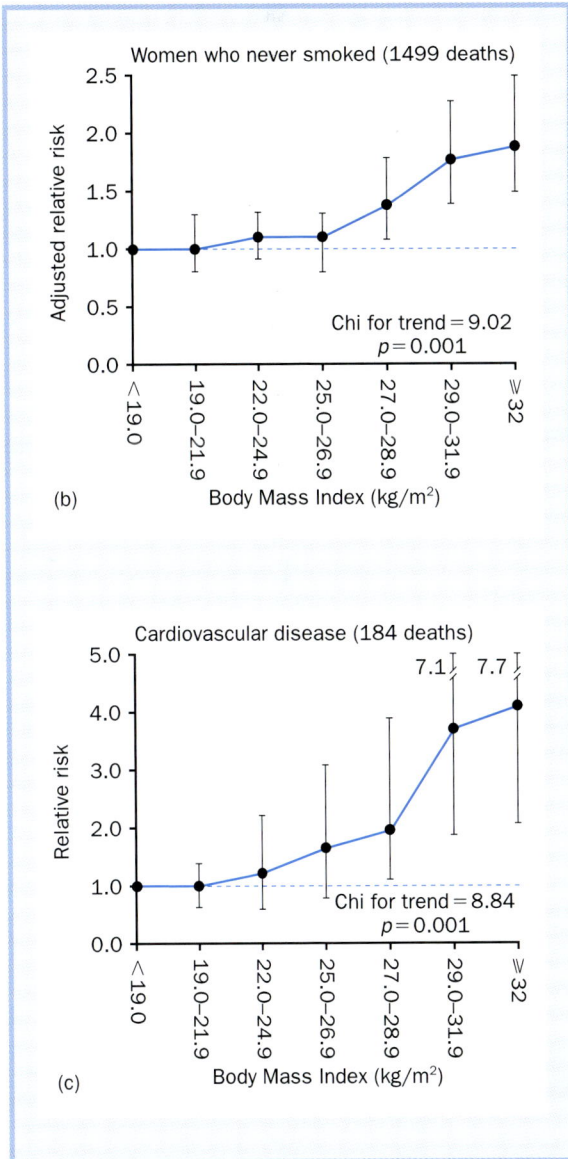

(b)

(c)

Figure 4.2
Data from the Nurses' Health Study showing (panel A) the relationship between obesity and overall mortality in all subjects. The relationships is stronger in those who do not smoke (panel B), presumably because of the facts that smoking induces weight loss both pharmacologically and pathologically. The relationship between obesity and cardiovascular mortality (panel C) is stronger than that for all-cause mortality, confirming obesity as a strong cardiovascular risk factor. Data from Manson et al.[9]

associations between mortality and body mass index (in all subjects and in nonsmokers only).

Cardiovascular disease and co-morbidities of obesity

Some of the co-morbidities are strong risk factors for cardiovascular disease. As indicated in Figure 4.1, obstructive sleep apnoea, dyslipidaemia, hypertension and diabetes mellitus each predispose to cardiovascular disease. These are discussed in separate chapters.

Sleep apnoea and cardiovascular disease

As discussed more fully in Chapter 6, obesity is strongly associated with obstructive sleep apnoea and related causes of nocturnal hypoventilation. These conditions strongly predispose to cardiovascular disease.

Obesity-induced diabetes and cardiovascular disease

As discussed more fully in Chapter 2, obesity is commonly complicated by diabetes mellitus. The induction of insulin resistance by obesity is thought to be the major cause of diabetes in this situation. In epidemiological studies it is well established that subjects with mild elevations of blood glucose, who are not diabetic, have increased cardiovascular

mortality, but many of those analyses did not try to dissect the independent effects of obesity and hyperglycaemia on cardiovascular mortality. Diabetes mellitus is associated with an increase in cardiovascular mortality of about 3-fold in men and about 5-fold in women, irrespective of obesity.[10]

Obesity-related hypertension

Obesity is strongly associated with hypertension. About 55% of patients in hypertension clinics are obese and about 50% of morbidly obese patients are hypertensive.[11] Having said that, conventionally-sized cuffs are usually too small for obese subjects which causes overestimation of blood pressure. This can lead to patients being mislabelled as hypertensive.

The cause of hypertension in obesity is not fully understood but several features of obesity are potentially capable of raising blood pressure (Table 4.2). The increased body mass of obesity requires an increase in oxygen consumption and cardiac output. In simple obesity, both oxygen consumption and cardiac output typically increase in proportion to body surface area.[12] The increase in cardiac output is achieved by several mechanisms including increased preload and increased cardiovascular sympathetic drive. Blood volume is increased in obesity in proportion to the increased body mass. Because blood volume increases with obesity proportionally

Table 4.2
Factors contributing to hypertension in obesity.

Factors arising from adipose tissue
- *Increased cortisone to cortisol conversion*
- *Increased leptin secretion*
- *Increased angiotensin release*

Factors arising from central (hypothalamic) abnormalities
- *Increased sympathetic nervous drive to vasculature*
- *Increased hypothalamo-pituitary-adrenal axis (HPA) activation*

Factors arising from other co-morbidities
- *Hyperinsulinaemia*
- *Hypoxia, especially at night*

Uncertain mechanism
- *Endothelial dysfunction*
- *Increased blood volume*
- *Reduced atrial naturetic peptide (ANF)*

Factors epidemiologically linked with obesity
- *Increased salt intake*
- *Lack of physical fitness*
- *Psychosocial stress*

Artefactual
- *Use of undersized manometer cuffs that mis-read blood pressure*

more than does cardiac output, even simple obesity is a volume expanded state.[12] This hypervolaemia increases preload on the heart.

Hormonal regulation of blood volume by atrial naturetic peptide may be abnormal in obesity. Adipose tissue converts cortisone to cortisol and the expanded adipose tissue mass of obesity may contribute to subtle changes in glucocorticoids that contribute to hypertension. Adipose tissue is believed to secrete factors such as angiotensinogen directly linked to increased hypertension, and leptin may also have a direct effect in inducing hypertension.[13] Sympathetic nervous system (SNS) vascular tone is increased in obesity, as reflected by increased urinary noradrenaline secretion, increased heart rate and reduced heart rate variability.[14] Endothelial function, as determined by post-ischaemic vasodilatation and intimal-media thickness, is abnormal in obesity.[15] Whether the endothelial abnormalities are attributable to the endocrine or SNS abnormalities mentioned above is not clear. In epidemiological studies, obese patients tend to have high salt intakes[16] and low levels of physical fitness, which are independently linked to hypertension.[17]

In summary, it would appear that obese subjects are prone to hypertension, but the mechanism(s) of this tendency is not clearly understood. It is likely that there are several mechanisms underlying the hypertension of obese subjects. Whether the mechanisms are the same in different obese patients remains to be established.

Clinical manifestations of obesity-related cardiovascular disease

Cardiovascular disease in obese subjects may have a variety of presentations. These include:

(1) Cardiomyopathies and heart failure
(2) Arrhythmias and sudden death
(3) Atherosclerotic coronary disease
(4) Venous thromboembolic disease

Clearly these presentations are not mutually exclusive, many patients may have more than one of these presentations. However, for simplicity, these different presentations will be discussed separately.

Cardiomyopathies

In this chapter the term cardiomyopathy will be used to mean the changes in cardiac morphology and function that occur unrelated to atherosclerotic coronary disease. Hypertrophic and dilated cardiomyopathies are common in obesity. In obese subjects there are commonly several possible causes for these changes. Thus diabetes, hypertension, nocturnal hypoxia and hypervolaemic states may co-exist. In milder cases, the patient will have a reduced cardiac reserve and hence limited exercise tolerance. More severe cases presenting clinically will usually present as heart failure. In the Framingham epidemiological study, heart failure was twice as common in obese patients as in lean.[5] Furthermore, in the lean subjects a specific cause for the heart failure (for example valve or alcohol) was identified in most subjects. Conversely in obese subjects, even histopathological studies can usually find no other specific cause of the heart failure (except obesity per se).[12]

Macroscopically there are marked changes in the hearts of obese subjects. As long ago as the 1930s, a series of autopsies was performed on patients dying of heart failure who were free of atherosclerotic coronary disease.[18] In this series, there was a relationship between body weight and cardiac weight. The increase in cardiac weight in obesity is partly due to fatty infiltration, but mostly due to increased mass of cardiac muscle and hypertrophy of myocardial cells. In a small proportion of cases, more florid fatty infiltration is seen, but the functional significance of this is uncertain.[19]

As indicated in Figure 4.3, a series of

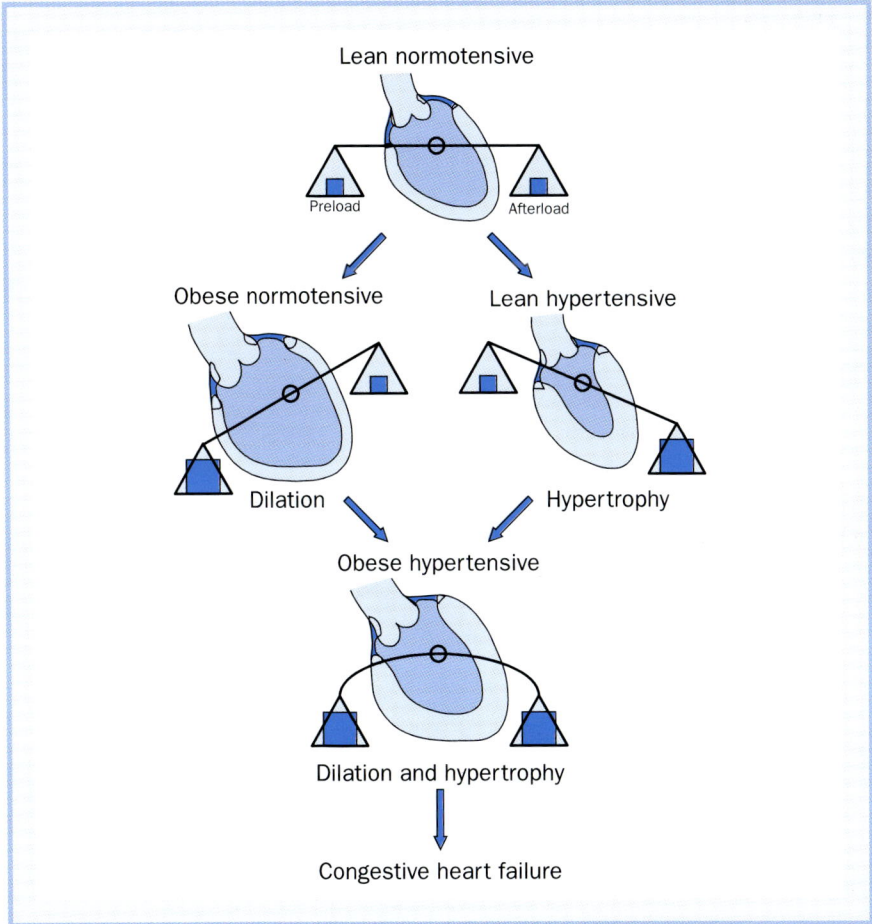

Figure 4.3
Effect of obesity and hypertension on cardiac structure. Adapted from Messerli FH.[20]

autopsies suggested that in subjects with 'pure' volume overload, dilated cardiomyopathy is more common, whilst in those with 'pure' pressure overload, hypertrophic changes are common.[20] Cardiac hypertrophy, whether related to dilation or not, is a bad prognostic feature and is particularly associated with subsequent sudden death.[21]

Functional abnormalities seen on echocardiography are common in obese subjects.[22] Even in simple obesity, cardiac stroke volume and pulse rate are increased in line with the hypervolaemic conditions mentioned above. Most morbidly obese patients with co-morbidities have cardiac dilation and hypertrophy demonstrable by echocardiography. ECG diagnosis of hypertrophy is more problematic because of the effect of thickening of the chest wall. Typically left ventricular mass increases with adiposity. Some studies suggest left ventricular mass index is proportional to BMI, others that it is more closely related to percentage of body weight over ideal weight. However, as the strain on the heart persists both impaired systolic function and diastolic function typically develop.[22]

Diastolic abnormalities are common in obesity. As the cardiac hypertrophy develops, ventricular compliance declines with impaired left ventricular filling. Obesity has been suggested as the single commonest cause of diastolic dysfunction, accounting for over 50% of the cases of diastolic dysfunction seen in a typical British district general hospital.[23]

Systolic dysfunction, including reduced ejection fraction, occurs later than diastolic problems in the progression of the typical obesity cardiomyopathy(ies). It has been clearly shown that the prevalence of reduced ejection fraction increases with time in obese subjects.

Recent echocardiographic studies have also suggested right heart abnormalities are common in morbid obesity, with marked abnormalities including dilatation and poor diastolic function.[24]

The valvular abnormalities that have been reported in obese subjects, who have used appetite suppressants such as fenfluramine and dexfenfluramine, are considered to be more related to the drugs than obesity, however the mechanism involved is unclear.[25]

The progression of left ventricular hypertrophy through diastolic and systolic abnormalities commonly presents as heart failure, but it may present as arrhythmias.

Arrhythmias and sudden death

Cardiovascular disease in obesity can present as arrhythmias. The most common change in the pulse of obese subjects is probably the increased pulse rate of two to five beats per minute reported in most studies of obesity.[12] On the resting ECG, a prolonged Q-T interval is an important predictor of more serious arrhythmias. Detailed electrocardiographic monitoring reveals changes in QTc intervals and dispersal. Power spectral analysis shows an increase in the high frequency elements of the spectra, reflecting an increase in the ratio of sympathetic activity to parasympathetic activity.[26] Such features can also be shown in subjects gaining weight.[27] Although none of these features are specific to obesity, they are unwelcome changes and are bad prognostic factors for the subsequent development of serious arrhythmias and sudden death.

The link between sudden death and obesity was famously recognized by Hippocrates.[12] More recent epidemiological studies, such as the Framingham, have repeated the finding and demonstrated that the relationship between obesity and sudden death is independent of conventional risk factors.[5,28]

The genesis of these arrhythmias may relate to the presence of co-morbidities such as diabetes, nocturnal hypoventilation and hypertension. Ischaemia (in obese or nonobese patients) is a primary cause of arrhythmias independent of these factors. Studies of subjects with obstructive sleep apnoea show frequent and often serious arrhythmias including ventricular tachycardias both at night and during the day (Chapter 6). However, in view of the power-spectral changes and increase in resting pulse, activation of the sympathetic nervous system is probably an important pathogenic mechanism in obesity-related arrhythmias.[29] Conversely, the strong relationship between left ventricular mass and serious arrhythmias (including sudden death) indicates the best clinical marker for patients at risk of arrhythmias is the size of the ventricle at echocardiography. Some post mortem studies have suggested that fatty infiltration of the heart increases the likelihood of fatal arrhythmia.[19] This finding has been especially implicated in the cause of death in younger patients, as has damage to the conducting system by fibrosis or cardiac hypertrophy.[28] Older patients dying suddenly are more likely to show atherosclerotic heart disease or dilated cardiomyopathy at post mortem.

Thus, although the main mechanism underlying these fatal arrhythmias may be sympathetic overactivity, the best way in clinical practice to identify those at risk would be to measure left ventricular mass (once obstructive sleep apnoea has been excluded). Sudden death is reported to be five times more common in subjects with left ventricular hypertrophy (compared to the general population).[12,30]

Sudden death may be a manifestation of arrhythmia or atherosclerotic heart disease.

Atherosclerotic coronary disease

Atherosclerosis is common in obese subjects and can be shown frequently at postmortem.[12] However, perhaps because of co-existing cardiomyopathy, or co-existing diabetes, or perhaps because of low levels of physical exercise, morbidly obese patients often do not present with a 'classic' history of exertional angina.

As for the other clinical presentations of heart disease in obesity, the frequent presence of underlying co-morbidities such as diabetes, hypertension and nocturnal hypoventilation may contribute to the clinical picture. In particular, diabetes may lead to 'silent' ischaemia as well as predisposing to arrhythmias.

Multiple factors contribute to accelerated atherosclerosis in obesity. They may be grouped into those related to insulin resistance, those related to pro-inflammatory cytokines and those related to thrombogenic tendency.

Insulin resistance

The insulin resistance syndrome (also known as syndrome X or pleurimetabolic syndrome), which includes hyperinsulinaemia, hypertriglyceridaemia, low HDL cholesterolaemia, hypertension and glucose intolerance, has been widely suggested as increasing cardiovascular mortality (Chapters 2 and 3). Reaven and others have pointed to the co-segregation of these factors in the general population.[31] Reaven's hypothesis is based upon the fact that insulin is a pleiotropic hormone, and that simultaneous problems with several of insulin's actions generate a syndrome of co-segregating

problems known as the insulin resistance syndrome. The actions of insulin that are thought to be involved in the genesis of the insulin resistance syndrome are its hypoglycaemic action, its anti-lipolytic action, its effect on liver VLDL secretion and its hypertensive effects. The insulin resistance syndrome hypothesis is that the failure of insulin's hypoglycaemic action causes glucose intolerance and hyperglycaemia (which is often not usually severe enough to be diabetes mellitus). An associated failure of insulin's anti-lipolytic action allows an increase in circulating concentrations of nonesterified fatty acids (NEFA).

It has been recognized for several decades that obesity causes multiple abnormalities of lipid metabolism. The increase in the adipose tissue mass may be directly relevant to these abnormalities.[32] Excess NEFA release from adipose tissue increases the rate of supply of NEFA into the circulation (R_a NEFA). This appears to cause the liver to increase VLDL secretion. About 30 years ago, Kissebah showed a strong relationship between R_a NEFA and the hepatic production rate of VLDL.[33]

Furthermore, in postprandial conditions, obese subjects show marked abnormalities of lipid metabolism, especially after a high fat load. Adipose tissue plays an important role in postprandial lipid metabolism. The enzyme lipoprotein lipase (LPL) is crucial in this situation, and adipose tissue is a major (perhaps even the most important) site of its synthesis. Adipose tissue exports LPL protein into the circulation from where other tissues may take up the enzyme. LPL is the rate-limiting step for clearance of circulating lipids. In the postprandial state circulating lipids include chylomicrons from exogenous lipid and endogenous VLDL. Studies have shown that in lean subjects, local clearance of circulating triglyceride increases during the postprandial period.[32,34]

Hypertriglyceridaemia is strongly associated with low HDL cholesterol concentrations, and adipose tissue LPL may play a direct role in this link. LPL acts on circulating lipoproteins to remove triglyceride from the particle. However, as triglyceride is removed from the core of the particle, there appear to be concomitant changes in the surface components. It has long been hypothesized that triglyceride clearance from VLDL particles and chylomicrons is linked to accumulation of cholesterol in HDL particles, presumably by direct transfer of surface cholesterol from VLDL and chylomicrons. By mechanisms which are not yet fully understood, the hypertriglyceridaemia/low HDL dyslipidaemia and its associated slow turnover of the VLDL pool alter the conformation of the LDL in the circulation. Subjects with this dyslipidaemia (including most obese individuals) have normal amounts of LDL, but the particles are small, dense LDL enriched with triglyceride. Low

HDL, small dense LDL, hypertriglyceridaemia forms a well-recognized lipid pattern which has been labelled the atherogenic lipoprotein profile.[35]

Thus obese subjects show a reduced LPL action (compared to lean subjects) as judged by triglyceride clearance, and also by interparticle transfer of apolipoprotein A-I and cholesterol. These defects in interparticle transfer may contribute directly to the formation of atherogenic remnants. This is the most likely candidate mechanism for the dyslipidaemia of obesity, which is especially relevant when fat loads are consumed.

Other aspects of the insulin resistance syndrome in obesity include hyperinsulinaemia provoked by hyperglycaemia and hyperinsulinaemia causing increased sympathetic nervous system activity which contributes to the hypertension part of the syndrome (as discussed above).

Pro-inflammatory cytokines

The most recent addition to the discussion of the links between obesity and atherosclerotic heart disease is the recognition that adipose tissue can secrete several pro-inflammatory cytokines.[13] Tumour necrosis factor-α (TNFα) is perhaps the best known of these cytokines, but although its concentrations are elevated in obesity, there is doubt as to whether it acts remotely from the adipose tissue rather than being a paracrine/autocrine agent. Interleukin-

6 (IL-6) does appear more like an adipose tissue product that can have systemic effects. Other adipose tissue products include IL-1β and IL-8. Each of these cytokines can contribute to a pro-atherogenic state in various ways. TNFα can increase NEFA levels, inhibit LPL and impair glucose tolerance. IL-6 can inhibit LPL, activate the HPA and increase liver secretion of clotting factors.

The quantitative importance of these pro-inflammatory cytokines to the risk of atherosclerotic heart disease remains to be established and, as yet, there are no therapeutic consequences that have come from their recognition.

Prothrombotic tendency (see also Chapter 5)

There is a well-recognized increased tendency to thrombosis in obesity.[36] This may manifest as deep venous thrombosis (DVT), venous insufficiency, superficial thrombophlebitis and pulmonary emboli. Obesity is a strong risk factor for each of these problems. Venous insufficiency following DVT is a considerable source of morbidity in obesity and accounts for a significant health economic burden. Fatal pulmonary emboli are an important and often preventable problem that are particularly seen in obese subjects during their postoperative course. The low level of cardiovascular fitness seen in obese subjects may well mask nonfatal pulmonary emboli and lead to a delay in presentation and diagnosis. Venous problems in obesity are caused by hydrostatic problems related to increased intra-abdominal pressure, by immobility and by changes in the clotting tendency seen in obesity.

The changes in the clotting tendency in obesity include increased plasma concentrations of fibrinogen, factors VII and VIII, von Willebrand factor and several other clotting factors. Conversely, there are reduced concentrations of anti-thrombotic factors such as plasminogen activator inhibitor-1 (PAI-1). In epidemiological studies, concentrations of these pro- and anti-thrombotic factors show correlations (positive and negative, respectively) with vascular disease.

The mechanisms for these changes in pro- and anti-thrombotic factor concentrations are not clear. Some workers suggest these are responses to hypertriglyceridaemia, others point to correlations with the waist to hip ratio. However, as with several other issues in obesity and cardiovascular disease, deconvoluting these co-segregating factors is difficult: at present we understand the correlations but are less sure of the causes.

Ethnic and gender issues

It is well known that different ethnic groups have different susceptibilities to the co-morbidities of obesity. South Asians have very high rates of both diabetes and the insulin resistance syndrome. This is associated with increased vascular disease. The relationship between obesity and these complications of obesity is preserved in this ethnic group, with the line between BMI and frequency shifted to the left. For this reason there is currently debate as to whether South Asians should be considered obese with a BMI of 27 kg/m^2. The thresholds for intervention in obese South Asians should be set lower than those for Caucasian populations. However, apart from the increased susceptibility to the adverse effects of obesity in this ethnic group, there is no reason to believe that their management should be different.

Afro-Caribbeans have an increased propensity to hypertension and an increased prevalence of obesity. However, again the basic relationship between obesity and the co-morbidity remains, as does the need to treat obesity.

Patients with polycystic ovary syndrome (PCOS) are a group in whom obesity is thought to be especially common. In these women, there is known to be an increased vascular risk, but again obesity exacerbates the problems of PCOS. Weight loss may be especially beneficial to women with PCOS since it can improve fertility and reduce the menstrual irregularity and hirsuteness of these patients.

None of these examples deny the relationship between obesity and its cardiovascular complications, but they do change the level at which treatment of obesity should be considered.

Management (Table 4.3)
Diagnosis

It is very important to identify those obese patients with mild, early cardiovascular disease and treat aggressively. If the treatment is delayed until it is clinically advanced, the patient is likely to be immobile and the probability of weight loss at that stage is very low. Similarly, progressive immobility will make patients worse candidates for invasive cardiological options, with their mortality rate becoming very high with immobility-related thrombotic and pulmonary complications.

Unfortunately, early recognition of significant cardiovascular symptoms may be difficult because of the patient's habitual low exercise level. Radiology (for example chest X-ray) and cardiac investigations (exercise ECG and transthoracic echocardiography) may lack diagnostic power in these patients. A high index of clinical suspicion is required.

Co-morbidities

As emphasized above, cardiovascular disease in obese subjects is usually accompanied by one or more co-morbidities (diabetes, hypertension, obstructive sleep apnoea). The

Table 4.3
Management of heart disease in obesity.

Assessment		
	(1)	Frequent blood pressure checks
	(2)	Screening for other reversible risk factors, lipid levels, diabetes, smoking
	(3)	Awareness of possible OSA
	(4)	Low threshold for special investigations for
		• Cardiomyopathy: chest X-ray, echocardiography
		• Arrhythmia: ECG monitoring
		• Ischaemic heart disease: ECG, radionucleide stress tests (exercise ECG rarely practicable)
General treatment	(1)	Weight loss
	(2)	Exercise
	(3)	Aggressive treatment of co-morbidities
		• Diabetes
		• Obstructive sleep apnoea (OSA)
	(4)	Treatment of other risk factors (smoking, cholesterol)
	(5)	Be aware of drugs likely to increase body weight: calcium antagonists, beta-blockers
	(6)	Consider aspirin
Specific treatment	(1)	Hypertension
		• ACE inhibitors
		• Thiazide diuretics
	(2)	Cardiomyopathy/Left ventricular hypertrophy (LVH)
		• ACE inhibitors
		• Loop diuretics
	(3)	Arrhythmias
		• Treat any underlying hypertension or LVH
		• Consider anti-coagulation
		• Conventional anti-arrhythmic medication
	(4)	Ischaemic heart disease
		• Treat any underlying hypertension or LVH
		• Conventional anti-anginal medication (will probably require beta-blockers)

treatment for these is discussed in other chapters, but the cardiac prognosis may depend upon the successful recognition and management of these co-morbidities.

General treatment

Weight loss and increasing physical exercise reverse the pro-atherogenic risk factors. Successful weight loss reverses nocturnal hypoventilation and reduces plasma volume hypertension, left ventricular hypertrophy and SNS vascular tone. Arrhythmias decrease after weight loss has been achieved. Likewise metabolic abnormalities such as glucose tolerance, dyslipidaemia, hyperinsulinaemia and pro-thrombotic clotting profile all improve. Significant benefits can be seen from a weight loss of 5–10 kg.[2]

The risk of sudden death does not disappear immediately when patients start to lose weight, indeed it may become more likely, being recognized in patients who have had gastric weight-reducing operations. Sudden death is also a reported complication of very-low-calorie diets. Whether this is because patients losing weight rapidly are prone to protein undernutrition, electrolyte abnormalities or micronutrient deficiency is unclear. However, rapid weight reduction stimulates an SNS response which may also contribute to the tendency to sudden death. The tendency to sudden death appears to be a feature of rapid weight loss situations rather than of more gradual changes.

There are also concerns about the effect of weight cycling, although these seem to be diminishing as studies are reported that distinguish between intentional and unintentional weight loss.[37]

Subjects with obesity and cardiac problems may benefit from exercise, but obviously graded exercise (preferably as part of a prescribed, supervised scheme) may be especially important in this group of subjects.

Aspirin and newer anti-platelet agents are valuable and should be prescribed as appropriate for these high-risk patients.

Hypertension

Weight loss, as well as salt restriction and exercise, will reduce hypertension in obese subjects. Studies typically show that 1 kg of weight loss will reduce systolic blood pressure by 1.6 mm Hg and diastolic by 1.3 mm Hg.[38] Pulse rate and circulating catecholamines will decrease with significant weight loss.

The drug treatment of hypertension in obese subjects is not significantly different from that in lean subjects, although agents known to cause weight gain (for example through fluid retention) should be prescribed with circumspection if a patient is attempting to lose weight. The demotivating effect of iatrogenic fluid retention should always be considered in a patient actively seeking weight loss. Nonpharmacological options for reducing blood pressure may be especially valuable in obese subjects. Obese subjects often consume a high-salt diet and restriction may be particularly beneficial. Regarding the pharmacological options for treating hypertension in obesity, there are probably more outcome data for diuretics than for other groups of drugs, mainly because these agents have been the most studied. Other than that the choice of anti-hypertensive agents for an individual obese patient involves similar considerations to those in lean subjects and includes ethnic background (for example Afro-Caribbeans may benefit from thiazides and calcium antagonists), co-morbidities (for example beta-blockers are especially indicated in angina or left ventricular hypertrophy and contra-indicated in asthma) and individual tolerance (for example erectile dysfunction). ACE inhibitors may be especially valuable because of their effect on left ventricular hypertrophy and their side-effect profile.

Cardiovascular drugs

In general, the pharmacotherapy of cardiovascular disease in obese subjects is similar to that in lean subjects. Thus cardiomyopathy is treated with loop diuretics and angiotensin converting enzyme inhibitors. Arrhythmias are treated with similar agents, although a search for the underlying cause of an arrhythmia in an obese patient is more likely to focus on alcohol consumption, nocturnal hypoventilation and pulmonary emboli. Angina is treated with conventional agents, and although beta-blockers may tend to increase weight slightly, they should not be withheld for this reason.

Summary

Cardiovascular disease is the major final common pathway by which co-morbidities of obesity kill the patient. The aetiology of cardiovascular disease in obese patients is often multifactorial. The patients may present late, at which stage treatment options may be reduced. Successful management requires a high index of suspicion for the existence of cardiovascular disease and underlying co-morbidities (for example OSA may only be recognized when the patient presents with heart failure or arrhythmia). In this way cardiovascular disease may be recognized early. Treatment requires attention to the heart, to the obesity per se and to the co-existing co-morbidities.

References

1   De Franzo RA, Ferrannini E, Insulin resistance, *Diabetes Care* (1991) **14**:173–94.

2   The Royal College of Physicians. Clinical management of overweight and obese patients: with particular reference to the use of drugs. (1998) 1–30. London: Royal College of Physicians

3   Powell KE , Pratt M, Physical activity and health: avoiding the short and miserable life, *Br Med J* (1996) **313**:126–7.

4   Garrison RJ, Higgins MW, Kannel WB, Obesity and coronary heart disease, *Curr Opin Lipidol* (1996) 7:199–202.

5   Hubert HB, Feinleib M, McNamara PM, Castelli WP, Obesity as an independent risk

factor for cardiovascular disease: a 26-year follow-up of participants in the Framingham Heart Study, *Circulation* (1983) 67:968–77.

6 Allison DB, Fontaine KR, Manson JE, Stevens J, VanItallie TB, Annual deaths attributable to obesity in the United States, *J Am Med Assoc* (1999) 282:1530–8.

7 Hu FB, Stampfer MJ, Manson JE et al, Trends in the incidence of coronary heart disease and changes in diet and lifestyle in women, *N Engl J Med* (2000) 343:530–7.

8 Seidell JC, Bouchard C, Visceral fat in relation to health: is it a major culprit or simply an innocent bystander? *Int J Obes Rel Metab Disord* (1997) 21:626–31.

9 Manson JE, Willett WC, Stampfer MJU, Body weight and mortality among women. *N Engl J Med* (1995) 333:677–85.

10 Fuller JH, Stevens LK, Wang S-L, International variations in cardiovascular mortality associated with diabetes mellitus: the WHO Multinational Study of Vascular Disease in Diabetes, *Ann Med* (1996) 28:319–22.

11 Sharma AM, Moeller T, Engeli S, Hypertension in obesity: its epidemiology, physiopathology and treatment efforts, *Dtsch Med Wochenschr* (1999) 124:1337–41.

12 Saltzman E, Benotti PN, The effects of obesity on the cardiovascular system. In: Bray GA, Bouchard C, James WPT, eds, *Handbook of Obesity* (New York: Marcel Dekker, 1997) 637–49.

13 Mohamed-Ali V, Pinkney JH, Coppack SW, Adipose tissue as an endocrine and paracrine organ, *Int J Obes Rel Metal Disord* (1998) 22:1145–58.

14 Esler M, Kaye D, Increased sympathetic nervous system activity and its therapeutic reduction in arterial hypertension, portal

hypertension and heart failure, *J Autonom Nerv Syst* (1998) 72:210–19.

15 Rocchini AP, Obesity and blood pressure regulation. In: Bray GA, Bouchard C, James WPT, eds, *Handbook of Obesity* (New York: Marcel Dekker, 1997) 677–95.

16 He J, Ogden LG, Vupputuri S, Bazzano LA, Loria C, Whelton PK, Dietary sodium intake and subsequent risk of cardiovascular disease in overweight adults, *JAMA* (1999) 282:2027–34.

17 Blair SN, Brodney S, Effects of physical inactivity and obesity on morbidity and mortality: current evidence and research issues, *Med Sci Sports Exercise* (1999) 31:S646–62.

18 Smith HL, Willius FA, Adiposity of the heart: a clinical and pathological study of one hundred and thirty-six obese patients, *Ann Int Med* (1933) 52:930–1.

19 Carpenter HM, Myocardial fat infiltration, *Am Heart J* (1962) 63:491–6.

20 Messerli FH, Cardiovascular effects of obesity and hypertension, *Lancet* (1982) i:1165–8.

21 Messerli FH, Hypertension, left ventricular hypertrophy, ventricular ectopy, and sudden death, *Am J Hypertens* (1993) 6:335–6.

22 Grossman E, Oren S, Messerli FH, Left ventricular filling in the systemic hypertension of obesity, *Am J Cardiol* (1991) 68:57–60.

23 Caruana L, Petrie MC, Davie AP, McMurray JJV, Do patients with suspected heart failure and preserved left ventricular function suffer from 'diastolic heart failure' or from misdiagnosis? A prospective descriptive study, *Br Med J* (2000) 321:215–19.

24 Bowles LJ, Timms A, Kepelman PG, Right ventricular abnormalities in obesity, European Congress of Obesity, Brussels 2001.

25 Gross SB, Appetite suppressants and cardiac

valvulopathy, Current clinical perspectives, *Adv Nurse Pract* (1999) 7:36–40.

26 Gao YY, Lovejoy JC, Sparti A, Bray GA, Keys LK, Partington C, Autonomic activity assessed by heart rate spectral analysis varies with fat distribution in obese women, *Obes Res* (1996) 4:55–63.

27 Arone LJ, Mackintosh R, Rosenbaum M, Leibel RL, Hirsch J, Autonomic nervous system activity in weight gain and weight loss. *Am J Phys* (1995) 269:R222–5.

28 Duflou J, Virmani R, Rabin I, Burke A, Farb A, Smialek J, Sudden death as a result of heart disease in morbid obesity, *Am Heart J* (1995) 130:306–13.

29 Rumantir MS, Vaz M, Jennings GL et al, Neural mechanisms in human obesity-related hypertension, *J Hypertens* (1999) 17:1125–33.

30 Messerli FH, Ketelhut R, Left ventricular hypertrophy: an independent risk factor. *J Cardiovasc Pharmacol* (1991) 17(Suppl 4):S59–66.

31 Reaven GM, The role of insulin resistance in human disease, *Diabetes* (1988) 37:1595–607.

32 Frayn KN, Coppack SW, Insulin resistance, adipose tissue and coronary heart disease, *Clin Sci* (1992) 82:1–8.

33 Kissebah AH, Alfarsi S, Adams PW, Wynn V, Role of insulin resistance in adipose tissue and liver in the pathogenesis of endogenous hypertriglyceridaemia in man, *Diabetologia* (1976) 12:563–71.

34 Coppack SW, Evans RD, Fisher RM et al, Adipose tissue metabolism in obesity: lipase action *in vivo* before and after a mixed meal, *Metabolism* (1992) 41:264–72.

35 Austin MA, King M-C, Vranizan KM, Krauss RM, Atherogenic lipoprotein phenotype. A proposed genetic marker for coronary artery disease risk, *Circulation* (1990) 82:495–506.

36 Blaszyk H, Wollan PC, Witkiewicz AK, Bjornsson J, Death from pulmonary thromboembolism in severe obesity: lack of association with established genetic and clinical risk factors, *Virchows Arch* (1999) 434:529–32.

37 Allison DB, Zannolli R, Faith MS et al, Weight loss increases and fat loss decreases all-cause mortality rate: results from two independent cohort studies, *Int J Obes Relat Metab Disord* (1999) 23:603–11.

38 Singh RB, Niaz MA, Bishnoi I, Singh U, Begum R, Rastogi SS, Effect of low energy diet and weight loss on major risk factors, central obesity and associated disturbances in patients with essential hypertension, *J Hum Hypertens* (1995) 9:355–62.

Obesity and abnormalities of haemostasis

Louise Bowles

5

Introduction

It is now generally accepted that the haemostatic system plays an important role in the pathogenesis of atherosclerotic plaques and their acute complications.[1–3] In the acute situation, plaque rupture is followed by vessel occlusion with thrombus and subsequent ischaemic damage. The rate of revascularization is crucial in limiting damage. Clearly, the haemostatic system plays an important role in this setting. Support has gathered for the idea that the coagulation system also has a role in the chronic disease process. Endothelial damage occurs after prolonged exposure to micro-thrombi and clot associated factors such as platelet-derived growth factor (PDGF), epidermal growth factor (EGF), and thrombin, which stimulate chemotaxis and proliferation of vascular smooth muscle cells, ultimately promoting the development of atherosclerosis. In addition, fibrin is a component of atherosclerotic plaques.[3] With this in mind, it seems logical to hypothesize that a pro-thrombotic environment and/or a situation where thrombus is not cleared effectively would predispose an individual to the development of atherosclerosis and its clinical sequelae.

Plasminogen activator inhibitor-1

Plasminogen activator inhibitors and cardiovascular disease

The fibrinolytic system is a complex system that is regulated by a balance between activators and inhibitors (Figure 5.1). Plasminogen activator inhibitor-1 (PAI-1) is the main inhibitor of fibrinolysis. PAI-1 binds to and inactivates tissue plasminogen activator (t-pa) and urokinase-like plasminogen activator (u-pa), the main activators of plasminogen. As PAI-1 levels increase, plasminogen activation is reduced and consequently fibrin accumulates. In this situation the balance is therefore in favour of thrombosis. PAI-1 has also been shown to have a local effect on the endothelium via activation of proteases and growth factors. Thus, high concentrations of PAI-1 are likely to favour the development of atherosclerosis and its acute complications. There is increasing evidence to support the hypothesis that high PAI-1 levels are associated with an increased risk of developing atherosclerosis. Atherosclerotic vessel walls contain higher concentrations of PAI-1 and PAI-1 mRNA than normal vessel walls, although it is not clear whether this relationship represents cause or effect.[4] Several cross-sectional studies have demonstrated high PAI-1 concentrations in subjects with coronary heart disease (CHD).[5,6] These results should, however, be interpreted with caution as episodes of cardiac ischaemia can result in transient increases in PAI-1 concentrations.[7]

Prospective studies are now available that provide important information on the prognostic value of PAI-1 levels in both healthy volunteers and those with CHD. In a study by Hamsten et al, PAI-1 levels were measured in 109 young survivors of myocardial infarction over a 3-year period.[8] Patients with CHD had higher levels of PAI-1 compared to matched controls. In addition, high PAI-1 levels were associated with an increased risk of re-infarction, even after adjusting for the degree of coronary disease and left ventricular dysfunction as well as for serum lipid concentrations. These findings have been supported by other published results. The Angina Prognosis Study in Stockholm (APSIS) reported that PAI-1 activity was independently predictive of myocardial infarction or cardiovascular death in men with angina.[9] In a recent study of 76 young male patients who had a myocardial infarction and underwent coronary angiography, high PAI-1 activity was associated with higher rates of disease progression, as assessed by repeat angiography after 5 years.[10] PAI-1 also appears to be predictive of cardiac events in subjects with no prior history of CHD. In a group of 78 healthy Swedish men and women, PAI-1 concentrations were higher in those volunteers who went on to develop a first myocardial

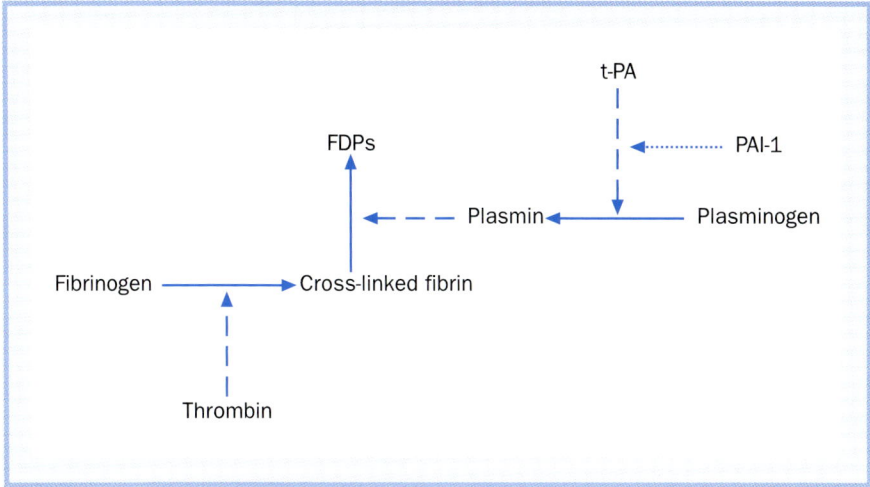

Figure 5.1
The Fibrinolytic system. FDPs, Fibrinogen degradation products; PAI-1, plasminogen activator inhibitor-1; dashed arrows indicate activation; dotted arrows indicate inhibition.

infarct compared to PAI-1 levels in a control group of 156 matched subjects.[11] In this study, PAI-1 did not remain predictive after adjusting for traditional cardiovascular risk factors. The relationship between PAI-1 and cardiovascular risk factors was explored in the European Concerted Action on Thrombosis and Disabilities (ECAT) study. In this study, PAI-1 and a number of other fibrinolytic variables were measured in 3,043 patients with angina, over a 2-year period.[12,13] PAI-1 antigen and activity were positively associated

with the development of acute myocardial infarction and sudden death. However, after adjusting for confounding variables that form part of the insulin resistance syndrome, namely body mass index (BMI), triglycerides and HDL cholesterol concentrations, this association disappeared. The prognostic value of PAI-1 seems to be related to its association with the insulin resistance syndrome. This is of considerable relevance when assessing a patient with abdominal obesity.

Plasminogen activator inhibitors and obesity

Information from a number of cross-sectional studies suggests that PAI-1 is positively correlated with BMI.[14–18] Swedish investigators measured PAI-1 activity in 260 volunteers, aged between 30 and 60 years and found a correlation between PAI-1 and BMI in both men and women.[14] In the North Sweden MONICA study of 1,558 men and women aged between 25 and 64 years, haemostatic factors including PAI-1 activity were measured and found to be correlated with anthropometric measures, as well as various other metabolic indices and blood pressure.[15] This study demonstrated a strong correlation between PAI-1 and BMI. An association between PAI-1 and adiposity has also been demonstrated in children aged between 7 and 11 years.[18] It would seem that even in early childhood, obesity is associated with unfavourable changes in haemostatic factors. Landin et al reported increased PAI-1 concentrations in obese subjects when compared to a control group of lean women.[19] The investigators went on to show that PAI-1 concentrations were significantly higher in 10 obese women with a high waist-to-hip ratio (WHR), compared to 10 carefully matched obese women with a low WHR. Overall, PAI-1 correlated more strongly with WHR than with BMI. WHR is an indirect measure of visceral fat and subsequent studies have

confirmed a strong association between PAI-1 and WHR. For example, Vague et al noted an association between WHR and PAI-1 concentrations in 51 pre-menopausal non-diabetic obese women.[20] Exploring this relationship further, investigators have used computerized tomography (CT) to quantify visceral fat mass and have correlated findings with PAI-1 concentrations. Shimomura et al used CT at the level of the umbilicus to assess the degree of visceral and subcutaneous fat in 61 obese and 40 lean men and women.[21] The mean BMI of the obese group was $31 \pm 5 \text{kg/m}^2$ compared to $23 \pm 2 \text{kg/m}^2$ in the lean group. For obese male and female volunteers, the investigators found a strong and significant correlation between visceral fat mass and PAI-1 concentrations ($r = 0.32$, $p < 0.02$). In contrast, PAI-1 was not correlated with subcutaneous fat mass. The investigators did not report the relationship of PAI-1 to total fat mass. Similar results were obtained in lean volunteers. In a study of 52 men, aged 38 years, CT was used to estimate visceral fat mass.[22] The investigators found that men with a visceral fat mass above the median value had significantly higher PAI-1 activity (19.2 ± 2.4 vs. $8.5 \pm 1.6 \text{ AU/ml}$ $p < 0.001$). Janand-Delenne et al studied 42 pre-menopausal women and confirmed a strong correlation between PAI-1 and visceral fat mass estimated by CT at the level of L3-L4 ($r = 0.533$ $p < 0.001$).[23] This association was independent of metabolic variables. Additionally, PAI-1 activity was related to total fat mass. It was calculated that visceral adipose tissue mass explained 28% of the variance in PAI-1 activity.

It is now well established that the distribution of adipose tissue as well as the amount of body fat are important determinants of morbidity and mortality. Subjects with a predominance of abdominal fat have a higher incidence of cardiovascular disease.[24] It is possible that the elevated PAI-1 levels associated with abdominal obesity may partly explain the increased risk of thrombosis in these subjects. From the evidence presented, it is clear that a strong relationship exists between PAI-1 concentrations and fat mass, particularly visceral fat mass, in humans. However, this association does not necessarily imply causality.

Plasminogen activator inhibitors and obesity: the link to the insulin resistance syndrome

In the insulin resistance syndrome, central obesity, hypertension, hyperinsulinaemia, hypertriglyceridaemia, and low HDL cholesterol concentrations are associated with an increased risk of developing atherosclerosis.[25] PAI-1 is positively correlated with each of the variables that make up the insulin resistance syndrome.[12,13] In addition to the correlation between PAI-1 and measures of adiposity, a clear association has been described between PAI-1 and fasting insulin

concentrations in a number of different subject groups, including the obese.[16,19,20,26–30] For example, The Insulin Resistance Atherosclerosis Study (IRAS) reported a strong and independent relationship between PAI-1 and insulin in subjects with normal glucose tolerance ($r = 0.42$), impaired glucose tolerance ($r = 0.38$) and type 2 diabetes ($r = 0.26$).[28] In obese subjects, Landin et al reported a positive correlation between PAI-1 levels and fasting glucose and insulin concentrations.[19] This study also demonstrated a correlation between PAI-1 and insulin sensitivity measured by euglycemic clamp technique. In a smaller study by Potter van Loon et al, PAI-1 antigen was significantly correlated with peripheral insulin resistance estimated by hyperinsulinaemic euglycemic clamp technique.[30] Using multiple regression analysis, the investigators demonstrated that the association between fasting insulin and PAI-1 antigen was secondary to the association between PAI-1 antigen and insulin resistance. PAI-1 is also correlated with triglyceride levels[13,15] as well as systolic and diastolic blood pressure.[13–15] The Biguanides and the Prevention of the Risk of Obesity (BIGPRO) study showed that patients with an increasing number of features of insulin resistance syndrome had higher PAI-1 levels.[31]

The evidence seems to point towards a strong relationship between PAI-1 and the insulin resistance syndrome and it may be that high PAI-1 levels contribute to the increased risk of atherosclerosis seen in this condition.

Interventional studies

The effect of weight loss on PAI-1 concentrations strengthens the hypothesis that there is a causal relationship between fat mass and PAI-1 levels. Intervention studies also allow us to determine what role the environment has on PAI-1 concentrations, as opposed to genetic predisposition.

In 1992, Folsom et al studied the effect of weight loss in 178 moderately overweight men and women.[32] The average BMI before weight loss was 31 kg/m². Subjects were randomly assigned to receive dietary counselling or to enter a control group for 6 months. In the treatment groups, the net weight loss was 9.4 kg in men and 7.4 kg in women. Weight reduction was associated with a reduction in PAI-1 antigen of 31% compared to baseline. Reductions in PAI-1 antigen were more strongly correlated with changes in anthropometric variables than with changes in fasting insulin or triglyceride concentrations, suggesting that weight loss per se is a more important determinant of PAI-1 concentrations than improvements in insulin resistance. Marckmann et al studied 43 subjects with a mean BMI of 35.5 kg/m².[33] Weight loss was achieved by energy-restricted diets for a 6-month period. After this time the average BMI fell to 30.3 kg/m². This was

associated with a fall in PAI-1 concentration of 34% compared to baseline levels. Several studies have demonstrated falls in PAI-1 levels associated with weight loss achieved by a variety of different methods such as, very-low calorie diets,[33] gastric surgery[34] and more moderate degrees of energy restriction.[35] Overall, it seems that even modest degrees of weight loss have beneficial effects on fibrinolysis.

Reductions in PAI-1 concentration have been correlated with a reduction in visceral fat mass, as measured by CT, but not with a fall in total fat mass, subcutaneous fat mass, insulin or triglyceride levels.[36] These results support an independent link between PAI-1 and visceral fat. The relationship between visceral fat mass and PAI-1 has been examined in a study of 50 subjects with a mean BMI of 31.3 ± 4.5 kg/m² in women and 30.5 ± 2.2 kg/m² in men.[37] Subjects received a calorie-controlled diet for 13 weeks. Magnetic resonance imaging (MRI) was used to record visceral and subcutaneous fat mass changes. Before weight loss, visceral fat mass was significantly and independently correlated with PAI-1 in men. In contrast to previous reports, this relationship was not demonstrated in women. After 13 weeks, the mean BMI fell by 4.3 ± 1.4 kg/m² in women and 3.9 ± 1.0 kg/m² in men. This weight loss was accompanied by a significant reduction in visceral fat mass and PAI-1. Changes in visceral fat mass were correlated to changes in

PAI-1 in women ($r = -0.43$; $p < 0.05$) but not in men ($r = -0.01$: ns). The association in women disappeared after correction for total fat mass. These results question the hypothesis that visceral fat mass is a major and independent determinant of PAI-1 and underline the need to examine each gender separately in metabolic and haemostatic studies.

In the BIGPRO study, obese non-diabetic subjects were randomly assigned to either Metformin or placebo treatment for 1 year.[31] PAI-1 activity and antigen declined by a similar extent in the treatment and control groups. This reduction appeared to be related to a fall in body weight rather than treatment with Metformin. This suggests that weight loss per se and not improvements in insulin sensitivity are a more important determinant of changes in PAI-1.

Regulation of plasminogen activator inhibitor-1 production

Research has been directed at explaining the molecular mechanisms responsible for elevated concentrations of PAI-1 in obesity and the insulin resistance syndrome. PAI-1 is produced primarily from the liver but also from a variety of other sources including endothelial cells and adipose tissue. Results from animal and human studies suggest that adipose tissue may be an important source of PAI-1, particularly in models of obesity. In

1991, Sawdey and Loskutoff were the first to demonstrate that PAI-1 mRNA was expressed in murine adipose tissue in relatively high concentrations.[38] PAI-1 mRNA levels are 4 to 5-fold higher in adipose tissue of genetically obese mice (ob/ob), compared to adipose tissue taken from lean controls.[39] In this model of obesity, increased PAI-1 concentrations seem to be secondary to increased production of PAI-1 by adipose tissue. PAI-1 is also produced by human adipose tissue at both the adipocyte and stromal levels in vitro, in addition to which, incubated visceral adipose tissue produces more PAI-1 antigen than subcutaneous adipose tissue.[40] Eriksson et al studied PAI-1 expression in adipose tissue samples taken from the abdominal wall of obese and lean volunteers.[41] The investigators demonstrated that PAI-1 production in adipose tissue taken from obese subjects was higher than that taken from lean controls. This increased PAI-1 production correlated with elevated PAI-1 activity. The evidence suggests that increased adipocyte production of PAI-1 is responsible for elevated concentrations in obese subjects. As fat mass increases, so does PAI-1 production.

Given the close correlation between PAI-1 and insulin, it has been postulated that insulin may have a role in controlling PAI-1 production. Early in vitro studies have demonstrated that in the human hepatocellular cell line Hep G2, PAI-1 antigen and activity are increased by insulin infusions at similar concentrations to that in the portal vein after a meal.[42,43] Production of other hepatic proteins was not altered and insulin did not increase PAI-1 production from endothelial cells. These results suggest that hepatocytes may be an important source of PAI-1, its production being modulated by insulin. In vivo studies looking at the effect of insulin on PAI-1 levels have produced some contradictory results. Infusions of insulin into lean mice increased PAI-1 mRNA expression 6 to 8-fold in epididymal fat.[39] In humans however, hyperinsulinaemia has not been correlated with a rise PAI-1 concentration in most studies.[44] However, Medvescek et al have reported a transitory increase in PAI-1 after an oral glucose load in obese and lean volunteers.[45] The peak in PAI-1 occurred 1 hour after the peak in insulin levels. It seems likely that acute changes in insulin concentrations do not alter PAI-1 expression, but the effect of chronic hyperinsulinaemia associated with insulin resistance remains unclear. By decreasing the number of insulin receptors in the HepG2 cell line, an insulin resistant state can be created.[46] If the cells are then stimulated by insulin, PAI-1 production increases. This model may be a more accurate reflection of the in vivo situation in humans. Alternatively, lipids may alter PAI-1 metabolism and indeed, VLDL increases PAI-1 secretion from endothelial cells in vitro.[47] In samples of human subcutaneous adipose

tissue, PAI-1 production correlates with fat cell volume and lipid content of the cells.[48] In this study, the investigators postulated that adipocyte PAI-1 production is increased in obesity as a result of stimulation of PAI-1 production from triglyceride-laden adipocytes.

Adipose tissue is a major source of tumour necrosis factor alpha (TNF-α). TNF-α is a pluripotent cytokine, produced mainly by macrophages. In addition to its role in immunity, TNF-α also plays a part in glucose and lipid metabolism.[49] Experimental evidence suggests that TNF-α is involved in mediating the metabolic consequences of obesity associated insulin resistance. For example, obese mice lacking TNF-α function do not develop the metabolic profile of an insulin resistant state.[50] TNF-α impairs insulin receptor intracellular signalling thereby leading to a state of insulin resistance.[51] Elevated adipose TNF-α concentrations are found in obese mice.[52] In lean mice, treatment with TNF-α increases PAI-1 mRNA expression in adipose tissue, as well as inducing PAI-1 expression in cultured 3T3-L1 cells, an adipocyte cell line.[53] Adipose tissue samples from obese subjects express more PAI-1 MRNA compared to lean controls.[54] Secretion of TNF-α and PAI-1 from human adipose tissue is correlated and the addition of an inhibitor to TNF-α synthesis, results in decreased PAI-1 synthesis.[55] Obesity is associated with elevated

TNF-α concentrations, which seem to be in part responsible for the development of an insulin resistant state. Additionally, TNF-α may have a role in regulating the expression of PAI-1 in adipose tissue.

Transforming growth factor-β (TGF-β) concentrations are higher in obese mice compared to lean controls.[56] Infusions of TGF-β induce PAI-1 mRNA expression in mouse adipose tissue.[38,56] TGF-β also stimulates PAI-1 gene expression in cultured human adipocytes.[38] There is evidence that TNF-α has a role in the regulation of TGF-β expression.[53]

Elevated PAI-1 in obesity may be secondary to chronic elevations in TNF-α, TGF-β, insulin and possibly other factors, which stimulate increased PAI-1 production from adipose tissue. The complex relationship between adipose tissue, PAI-1 and cytokines has not yet been fully explained.

Fibrinogen

Fibrinogen and cardiovascular disease

Fibrinogen is now considered an important predictor of CHD and future cardiovascular events and may have a direct role in the atherosclerotic process.[57–60] Fibrinogen stimulates smooth muscle proliferation and migration, is a component of atherosclerotic plaques, promotes platelet aggregation and is a major contributor to blood viscosity. Increased fibrinogen levels contribute directly to a procoagulant state thereby favouring the development of atherosclerosis. Alternatively, because fibrinogen is an acute phase protein, high concentrations may simply reflect the inflammatory state associated with atherosclerosis.

The importance of fibrinogen concentrations in predicting future cardiovascular events was first demonstrated in The Northwick Park Heart Study.[57] In this study 1,511 men aged between 40 and 64 years were followed up for 10 years. Those people with pre-existing CHD were not excluded. The study demonstrated that a fibrinogen level in the upper third of the normal range increased the risk of CHD by 3-fold compared to those in the lower third. A plasma fibrinogen level of one standard deviation from the mean increased the risk of a first ischaemic event by 84% over the next 5 years. This association was independent of other traditional risk factors. Ernst and Resch performed a meta-analysis of six prospective epidemiological studies looking at the association between plasma fibrinogen and cardiovascular disease.[58] The summary odds ratio was estimated to be 2.3 (95% CI, 1.9–2.8). There is now strong evidence to support the link between fibrinogen and atherosclerosis and this association appears to be independent of other traditional risk factors.

Fibrinogen and obesity

Several large epidemiological studies have demonstrated that fibrinogen is correlated with both BMI and WHR.[59–65] Some investigators have seen this association in both men and women,[63] while others have found statistically significant results in women only.[60,64]

In the Scottish Heart Health Study multivariate analysis showed that fibrinogen was positively associated with BMI, although the association was weaker in men compared to women.[63] In the third Glasgow MONICA survey, 746 men and 816 women were randomly sampled to establish associations between certain haemostatic factors and risk factors for cardiovascular disease.[64] In this study fibrinogen was correlated with BMI in women but not in men. Likewise in the Framingham study fibrinogen concentrations increased with measures of adiposity in women but not in men.[60] Krobot et al examined the relationship between fibrinogen levels and various other cardiovascular risk factors in 4,434 subjects.[62] Fibrinogen was positively correlated with BMI and WHR in men and women. In men the relationship between fibrinogen and WHR was stronger than the relationship between fibrinogen and BMI. The opposite was true for women. In the PRIME Study, fibrinogen and a number of other haemostatic variables were measured in 10,500 men.[61] Fibrinogen was more strongly correlated with WHR than BMI. These results demonstrate the importance of central obesity, which is more common in male subjects, and emphasize the fact that the mechanisms controlling production of certain haemostatic factors differ between men and women.

Interventional studies

The association between fibrinogen and obesity is strengthened by results of interventional studies that have examined the effect that weight loss has on fibrinogen concentrations. A number of studies have shown that weight loss is accompanied by a reduction in fibrinogen concentration.[33,34,65,66] In the Northwick Park Heart study, 1,725 men from the original study were re-examined. Results from the study showed a 0.17% change in fibrinogen concentration per unit change in BMI.[65] Further studies have examined the effect of intentional weight loss in obese subjects. For example, obese subjects on a low calorie diet experienced a 6% decline in fibrinogen concentrations.[33] A reduction in fibrinogen from 3.5 to 2.8 g/l accompanied weight loss of 64 kg 1 year after gastric surgery was performed as treatment for morbid obesity.[34] However, there are some conflicting results.[31,32,67,68] For example, Folsom et al reported no net change in fibrinogen concentrations with weight loss of 9.4 kg in overweight men and women.[32] In the

BIGPRO study fibrinogen concentrations fell regardless of weight loss.[31] Mechanisms controlling fibrinogen production are likely to be complex.

Fibrinogen and insulin resistance: is there a link?

The link between fibrinogen and the parameters that make up the insulin resistance syndrome is more tenuous than the link between PAI-1 and these metabolic variables. A number of epidemiological studies have produced conflicting results. For example, some investigators have reported no relationship between insulin and fibrinogen levels[15,18] whilst other studies have reported an association.[13,22,69,70] In the Framingham Offspring study, insulin levels and oral glucose tolerance tests were recorded in 1,331 men and 1,631 women aged between 26 and 82 years.[71] In those women with normal glucose tolerance tests, mean levels of fibrinogen increased across fasting insulin quintiles. In those subjects with impaired glucose tolerance, there was no increase in fibrinogen concentrations with increasing fasting insulin levels. In contrast, a study examining the relationship between fibrinogen and metabolic abnormalities of the insulin resistance syndrome has shown that as the number of metabolic abnormalities increase, fibrinogen levels also increase.[72] In this study, after multivariate analysis was performed,

fibrinogen was shown to be significantly and independently correlated with metabolic features in the insulin resistance syndrome. The DESIR (data from an epidemiological study on insulin resistance) study group reported results showing that fibrinogen concentrations in men and women are positively associated with fasting insulin and insulin resistance as measured by HOMA-IR (Homeostasis Model Assessment for Insulin Resistance).[70] The relationship was stronger in women than in men. In the Prime study, investigators noted that the insulin resistant variables of BMI, WHR, triglyceride and HDL concentration, NIDDM and physical inactivity accounted for approximately 1% of the variance in fibrinogen concentrations. In contrast, these same variables explained 24% of the variance in PAI-1 concentrations.[61]

The investigators in these studies have all used different methodologies, particularly when recording insulin resistance, and this may in part account for the contradictory results. Overall, however, it does seem that the relationship between fibrinogen and insulin resistance is stronger in women than in men.[70,71] However, it is likely that the relationship between fibrinogen and insulin resistance is not strong. Behavioural interventions such as weight loss improve insulin sensitivity. As already described, studies examining the effect of weight loss on fibrinogen concentrations have produced contradictory results, lending support to the idea that the relationship between fibrinogen and insulin resistance is at present uncertain.

Other haemostatic variables

In addition to PAI-1 and fibrinogen, a number of other haemostatic variables appear to be associated with an increased incidence of CHD.

The Northwick Park Heart Study showed Factor VII coagulant (VIIc) levels to be predictive of future coronary events, even after adjusting for fibrinogen, cholesterol and blood pressure.[57] The association was not as strong as for fibrinogen, but was stronger than for cholesterol. Although a number of studies have confirmed this relationship[73] conflicting results do exist.[61,68,74]

Haemophiliacs have a low incidence of CHD.[75] This has lead to the hypothesis that elevated factor VIII levels may be associated with a higher incidence of CHD. Prospective studies of subjects with and without vascular disease, have demonstrated an association between factor VIII levels and CHD. For example, Meade et al reported that an increase of one standard deviation in factor VIIIc raised the risk of fatal CHD by 28%.[76] This association has also been demonstrated in subjects with established atherosclerosis.[74] Von Willebrand factor (vWF) mediates platelet aggregation and is also an indicator of endothelial dysfunction. An association between vWF and CHD is now well

recognized. In the Northwick Park Heart Study, vWFAg was associated with fatal CHD.[76] vWF is also a predictor of coronary events in subjects with vascular disease.[74,77] High levels of vWF probably contribute to a prothrombotic state, but also reflect on-going endothelial damage in atherosclerotic vessels. As has already been discussed, impaired fibrinolysis is associated with a higher incidence of CHD. Studies linking t-PA activity and CHD have produced conflicting results. Hamsten et al found t-PA activity to be lower in patients with a myocardial infarction (MI), when compared to a matched group of controls.[5] However in the Physician's Health study, higher levels of t-PA antigen were strongly associated with the risk of future MI in apparently healthy men.[78]

How these haemostatic factors correlate with more traditional cardiovascular risk factors has been examined in a number of epidemiological studies. Factor VIIc levels are positively correlated with BMI in men and women.[61,64] A stronger relationship exists between factor VII and serum lipids, in particular triglyceride levels. Weight loss in obese and overweight subjects has been accompanied by significant decreases in factor VII levels in a number of studies.[32–34] In the MONICA study, factor VIIIc levels positively correlated with BMI in women but not in men,[64] whilst in the ARIC study, factor VIIIc was positively correlated with BMI and WHR in both men and women.[79] A positive correlation has been found between vWF and BMI in healthy men and women,[79] as well as in obese women with no history of CHD.[80] The Northern Sweden MONICA study found a significant correlation between t-pa activity and BMI in both men and women.[15] In women central obesity was a more important determinant of t-pa activity than obesity per se.[14,15] These associations do not necessarily imply causality. Further studies are needed to examine the effect of weight loss on these variables.

The association between obesity and venous thrombosis has been well documented.[81,82] This increased risk may also be partly mediated through changes in the haemostatic system. Deficiencies of the coagulation inhibitors antithrombin III, protein C and protein S are well-established risk factors for recurrent venous thrombosis. In addition, recent reports have highlighted the importance of high factor VIII levels in subjects with a first episode of deep vein thrombosis (DVT)[83] and in subjects with recurrent DVTs.[84]

The MONICA study found a statistically significant increase in protein C and S concentrations as BMI increased in both men and women.[64] Conlan et al also reported a correlation between protein C and BMI.[85] It would seem that both vitamin K dependent coagulation factors and vitamin K dependent coagulation inhibitors are correlated with changes in BMI. The rise in coagulation

inhibitors associated with obesity may reflect a compensatory response to activated coagulation and impaired fibrinolysis.

As the prevalence of obesity increases it becomes increasingly important to understand the pathophysiological consequences of increased fat mass. Clearly, obesity is associated with significant alterations in a number of haemostatic factors, which may help explain the increased incidence of thrombosis in these subjects.

References

1   Fuster V, Badimon L, Badimon J, Chesebro J, The pathogenesis of coronary artery disease and the acute coronary syndromes. Part 1. *N Engl J Med* (1992) 326:242–50.

2   Fuster V, Badimon L, Badimon J, Chesebro J, The pathogenesis of coronary artery disease and the acute coronary syndromes. Part 2. *N Engl J Med* (1992) 326:310–18.

3   Thompson WD, Smith EB. Atherosclerosis and the coagulation system. *J Path* (1989) 159:97–106.

4   Schneiderman J, Swadey MS, Keeton MR et al, Increased type 1 plasminogen activator inhibitor gene expression in atherosclerotic human arteries. *Proc Natl Acad Sci USA* (1992) 89:6998–7002.

5   Hamsten A, Wimna B, De Faire U, Blomback M, Increased plasma levels of a rapid inhibitor of tissue plasminogen activator in young survivors of myocardial infarction. *N Engl J Med* (1985) 313:1557–63.

6   Olofsson BO, Dahlen G, Nilsson TK, Evidence for increased levels of plasminogen activator

inhibitor and tissue plasminogen activator in plasma of patients with angiographically verified coronary artery disease. *Eur Heart J* (1989) **10**:77–82.

7   Sakata K, Kurata C, Kobayashi A et al, Plasminogen activator activity as a possible indicator of disease activity in rest angina with angiographically insignificant coronary artery stenosis. *Thromb Res* (1991) **63**:491–502.

8   Hamsten A, deFaire U, Walldius G, Plasminogen activator inhibitor-1 in plasma: risk factor for recurrent myocardial infarction. *Lancet* (1987) **2**:3–9.

9   Held C, Hjemdahl P, Rehnqvist N et al, Fibrinolytic variables and cardiovascular prognosis in patients with stable angina pectoris treated with Verapamil of Metoprolol. *Circulation* (1997) **95**:2380–6.

10 Bavenholm P, de Faire U, Landou C et al, Progression of coronary artery disease in young male post-infarction patients is linked to disturbances of carbohydrate and lipoprotein metabolism and to impaired fibrinolyitc function. *Eur Heart J* (1998) **19**:402–10.

11 Thogersen AM, Jansson J, Boman K, High plasminogen activator inhibitor and tissue plasminogen activator levels in plasma precede a first acute myocardial infarction in both men and women. *Circulation* (1998) **98**:2241–7.

12 Juhan–Vague I, Pyke SDM, Alessi MC et al, Fibrinolytic factors and the risk of myocardial infarction or sudden death in patients with angina pectoris. *Circulation* (1996) **94**:2057–63.

13 Juhan–Vague I, Thompson SG, Jespersen J, Involvement of the haemostatic system in the insulin resistance syndrome. A study of 1500 patients with angina pectoris. *Arterioscler Thromb* (1993) **13**:1865–73.

14 Sundell IB, Nilsson TK, Ranby M, Hallmans G, Hellsten G, Fibrinolytic variables are related to age, sex blood pressure, and body build measurements: a cross-sectional study in Norsjo, Sweden. *J Clin Epidemiol* (1989) **42**:719–23.

15 Eliasson M, Evrin PE, Lundblad D, Fibrinogen and fibrinolytic variables in relation to anthropometry, lipids and blood pressure. The Northern Sweden MONICA study. *J Clin Epidemiol* (1994) **47**:513–24.

16 Vague P, Juhan-Vague I, Aillaud MF, Badier C, Viard R, Alessi MC, Collen D, Correlation between fibrinolytic activity, plasminogen activator inhibitor level, plasma insulin and relative body weight in normal and obese subjects. *Metabolism* (1986) **35**:250–3.

17 Vague P, Juhan-Vague I, Chabert V, Alessi MC, Atlan C, Fat distribution an plasminogen activator inhibitor activity in non-diabetic obese women. *Metabolism* (1989) **38**:913–15.

18 Ferguson MA, Gutin B, Owens S, Litaker M, Tracy RP, Allison J, Fat distribution and haemostatic measures in obese children. *Am J Clin Nutr* (1998) **67**:1136–40.

19 Landin K, Stigendal L, Eriksson E, Krotkiewski M, Risberg B, Tengborn L, Smith U. Abdominal obesity is associated with an impaired fibrinolytic activity and elevated plasminogen activator inhibitor-1. *Metabolism* (1990) **39**:1044–8.

20 Vague P, Juhan-Vague I, Chabert V et al, Fat distribution and plasminogen activator inhibitor activity in non-diabetic obese women. *Metabolism* (1989) **9**:913–15.

21 Shimomura I, Funahashi T, Takahashi M et al, enhanced expression of PAI-1 in visceral fat: possible contributor to vascular disease in obesity. *Nat Med* (1996) **7**:800–3.

22 Cigolini M, Targher G, Bergamo Andreis IA et al, Visceral fat accumulation and its relation to plasma haemostatic factors in healthy men. *Arterioscler Thomb* (1996) **16**:368–74.

23 Janand-Delenne B, Chagnaud C, Raccah D, et al. Visceral fat as a main determinant of plasminogen activator inhibitor 1 level in women. *Int J Obesity* (1998) **22**:312–17.

24 Larsson B, Svardsudd K, Welin et al, Abdominal adipose tissue distribution, obesity and risk of cardiovascular disease and death. 13-year follow-up of participants in the study of men born in 1913. *BMJ* (1984) **288**:1401–4.

25 Reaven GM. Role of insulin resistance in human disease. *Diabetes* (1988) **37**:1595–607.

26 Juhan-Vague I, Roul C, Alessi MC et al, Increased plasminogen activator inhibitor activity in non-insulin dependent diabetic patients - the relationship with plasma insulin. *Thromb Haemost* (1989) **61**:370–3.

27 McGill JB, Schneider DJ, Arfken CL et al, Factors responsible for impaired fibrinolysis in obese subjects and NIDDM patients. *Diabetes* (1994) **43**:104–9.

28 Festa A, D'Aostino R, Mykkanen L et al, Relative contribution of insulin and its precursors to fibrinogen and PAI-1 in a large population with different states of glucose tolerance. The Insulin Resistance Atherosclerosis Study. (IRAS) *Arterioscl Thromb* (1999) **19**:562–8.

29 Juhan-Vague I, Alessi MC, Vague P. Increased plasma plasminogen activator inhibitor 1 levels. A possible link between insulin resistance and atherothrombosis. *Diabetologia* (1991) **34**:457–62.

30 Potter van Loon BJ, Kluft C, Radder JK et al, The cardiovascular risk factor plasminogen activator inhibitor type 1 is related to insulin resistance. *Metabolism* (1993) **42**:945–9.

31 Charles MA, Mornage P, Eschwege E et al, Effect of weight change and Metformin on fibrinolysis and the von Willebrand factor in obese non-diabetic subjects: the BIGPRO

Study. Biguanides and the prevention of the risk of obesity. *Diabetes Care* (1998) **21**:1967–72.

32 Folsom AR, Qamhieh HT, Wing RR et al, The impact of weight loss on plasminogen activator inhibitor, factor VII and other haemostatic factors in moderately overweight adults. *Arterioscler Thromb* (1993) **13**:162–9.

33 Marckmann P, Toubro S, Astrup A, Sustained improvement in blood lipids, coagulation and fibrinolysis after major weight loss in obese subjects. *Eur J Clin Nutr* (1998) **52**:329–33.

34 Primrose JN, Davies JA, Prentice CRM et al, Reduction in factor VII, fibrinogen and plasminogen activator inhibitor-1 activity after surgical treatment for morbid obesity. *Thromb Haemost* (1992) **68**:396–9.

35 Calles-Escandon J, Ballor D, Harvey-Beriono J et al, Amelioration of the inhibition of fibrinolysis in elderly, obese subjects by moderate energy intake restriction. *Am J Clin Nutr* (1996) **64**:7–11.

36 Janand-Delenne B, Chagnaud C, Raccah D et al, Visceral fat as a main determinant of plasminogen activator inhibitor 1 level in women. *Int J Obesity* (1998) **22**:312–17.

37 Kockx M, Leenen R, Seidell J et al, Relationship between visceral fat and PAI-1 in over weight men and women before and after weight loss. *Thromb Haemost* (1999) **82**:1490–6.

38 Sawdey MS, Loskutoff DJ, Regulation of murine type 1 plasminogen activator inhibitor gene expression in vivo. Tissue specificity and induction by lipopolysaccharide, tumour necrosis factor-alpha and transforming growth factor-beta. *J Clin Invest* (1991) **88**:1346–53.

39 Samad F, Loskutuoff DJ, Tissue distribution and regulation of plasminogen activator inhibitor-1 in obese mice. *Mol Med* (1996) **2**:568–82.

40 Alessi MC, Peiretti F, Morange P et al, Production of plasminogen activator inhibitor-1 by human adipose tissue. Possible link between visceral fat accumulation and vascular disease. *Diabetes* (1991) **46**:860–7.

41 Eriksson P, Reynisdottir S, Lonnqvist F et al, Adipose tissue secretion of plasminogen activator inhibitor-1 in non-obese and obese individuals. *Diabetologia* (1998) **41**:65–71.

42 Alessi MC, Juhan-Vague I, Kooistra T et al, Insulin stimulates the synthesis of plasminogen activator inhibitor 1 by the human hepatocellular cell line Hep G2. *Thromb Haemost* (1988) **60**:491–4.

43 Kooistra T, Bosma P, Tons H et al, Plasminogen activator inhibitor-1: Biosynthesis and mRNA levels are increased by insulin in cultures hepatocytes. *Thromb Haemost* (1989) **62**:723–8.

44 Grant PJ, Kruithof EKO, Felley CP et al, Short-term infusions of insulin, triacylglycerol and glucose do not cause acute increases in plasminogen activator inhibitor-1 concentrations in man. *Clin Sci* (1990) **79**:513–16.

45 Medvescek M, Keber D, Stegnar M, Borovnica A. Plasminogen activator inhibitor-1 response to a carbohydrate meal in obese subjects. *Fibrinolysis* (1990) **4**:89–90.

46 Anfosso F, Chomiki N, Alessi MC et al, Plasminogen activator inhibitor–1 synthesis in the hepatoma cell line HepG2. Metformin inhibits the stimulating effect of insulin. *J Clin Invest* (1993) **5**:2185–93.

47 Mussoni L, Maderna F, Camera M et al, Atherogeneic lipoproteins and release of plasminogen activator inhibitor-1 (PAI-1) by endothelial cells. *Fibrinolysis* (1990) **2** (suppl):79–81.

48 Eriksson P, Reynisdottir S, Lonnqvist F et al,

Adipose tissue secretion of plasminogen activator inhibitor-1 in non-obese and obese individuals. *Diabetologia* (1998) **41**:65–71.

49 Grunfield C, Feingold KR. The metabolic effects of tumour necrosis factor and other cytokines. *Biotherapy* (1991) **3**:143–58.

50 Uysal KT, Wiesbrock SM, Marino MW, Hotamisligil GS. Protection from obesity-induced insulin resistance in mice lacking TNF-α function. *Nature* (1997) **389**:610–14.

51 Hotamisligil GS, Murray DL, Choy LN, Spiegelman BM, TNF-α inhibits signalling from insulin receptor. *Proc Natl Acad Sci USA* (1994) **91**:4854–8.

52 Hotamisligil GS, Shargill NS, Spiegelman BM. Adipose tissue expression of tumour necrosis factor-alpha: a direct role in obesity-linked insulin resistance. *Science* (1993) **259**:87–91.

53 Samad F, Yamamoto K, Loskutoff DJ. Distribution and regulation of plasminogen activator inhibitor 1 in murine adipose tissue in vivo. *J Clin Invest* (1996) **97**:37–46.

54 Hotamisligil GS, Arner P, Caro JF et al, Increased adipose tissue expression of tumour necrosis factor alpha in human obesity and insulin resistance. *J Clin Invest* (1995) **95**:2409–15.

55 Agostino G, Tonoli M, Deorsola B et al, PAI-1 release form human adipose tissue is stimulated by TNF-alpha. *Thromb Haemost* (1997) **suppl** 749(abstract).

56 Samad F, Yamamoto K, Pandey M, Loskutoff D, Elevated expression of transforming growth factor-beta in adipose tissue from obese mice. *Mol Med* (1997) **3**:37–48.

57 Meade TW, Brozovic M, Chakrabarti R, Haines AP, Imenson JD, Mellows S et al, Haemostatic function and ischaemic heart

disease: principal results of the Northwick Park Heart study. *Lancet* (1986) **2**:533–7.

58 Ernst E, Resch KL. Fibrinogen as a cardiovascular risk factor: A meta-analysis and review of the literature. *Ann Intern Med* (1993) **118**:956–63.

59 Folsom AR, Qamhieh HT, Flack JM et al, Plasma fibrinogen: levels and correlates in young adults. The Coronary Artery Risk Development in Young Adults (CARDIA) Study. *Am J Epidemiol* (1993) **138**:1023–36.

60 Kannel WB, Wolf PA, Castelli WP, d'Agostino RB, Fibrinogen and the risk of cardiovascular disease; The Framingham study. *JAMA* (1997) **258**:1183–6.

61 Scarabin PY, Aillaud MF, Amouyel P et al, Association of fibrinogen, factor VII and PAI-1 with baseline findings among 10,500 male participants in a prospective study of myocardial infarction. The Prime Study. *Thromb Haemost* (1998) **80**:749–56.

62 Krobot K, Hense HW, Cremer P et al, Determinants of plasma fibrinogen: relation to body weight, waist-to-hip ratio, smoking, alcohol, age and sex. *Arterioscler Thromb* (1992) **12**:780–8.

63 Lee AJ, Smith WCS, Lowe GDO, Turnstall-Pedoe H, Plasma fibrinogen and coronary risk factors: the Scottish Health study. *J Clin Epidemiol* (1990) **43**:913–19

64 Woodward M, Lowe GDO, Rumley A, Epidemiology of coagulation factors, inhibitors and activation markers: The third Glasgow MONICA survey II. Relationships to cardiovascular risk factors and prevalent cardiovascular disease. *Br J Haematol* (1997) **97**:785–97.

65 Meade TW, Imeson J, Stirling Y, The effects of changes in smoking and other characteristics on

clotting factors and the risk of ischaemic heart disease. *Lancet* (1987) **2**:986–8.

66 Luckx FH, Scheen AJ, Desaive C et al, Effects of gastroplasty on body weight and related biological abnormalities in morbid obesity. *Diabetes* (1998) **24**:355–61

67 Svendsen OL, Hassager C, Christiansen C et al, Plasminogen activator inhibitor–1, tissue type plasminogen activator and fibrinogen. Effect of dieting with or without exercise in overweight postmenopausal women. *Arterioscler Thromb* (1996) **16**:381–5.

68 Mahrabian M, Peter JB, Barnard RJ, Lusis AJ, Dietary regulation of fibrinolytic factors. *Atheroscler* (1990) **84**:25–32.

69 Folsom AR, Wu KK, Rosamond WD et al, Prospective study of haemostatic factors and incidence of coronary artery disease. *Circulation* (1997) **96**:1102–8.

70 Mennen LI, Balkau B, Charles MA et al, Gender differences in the relation between fibrinogen, tissue-type plasminogen activator antigen and markers of insulin resistance: effects of smoking. *Thromb Haemost* (1999) **82**:1106–11.

71 Meigs JB, Mittleman MA, Nathan DM et al, Hyperinsulinemia, hyperglycemia, and impaired haemostasis: the Framingham Offspring Study. *JAMA* (2000) **283**:221–8.

72 Imperatore G, Riccardi G, Iovine C et al, Plasma fibrinogen: a new factor of the metabolic syndrome. A population-based study. *Diabetes Care* (1998) **21**:2040–1.

73 Heinrich J, Balleisen L, Schulte H et al, Fibrinogen and factor VII in the prediction of coronary risk. Results from the PROCAM study in healthy men. *Arterioscler Thromb* (1994) **14**:54–9.

74 Cortellaro M, Boschetti C, Confrancesco E,

The PLAT study: haemostatic function in relation to atherothrombotic ischaemic events in vascular disease patients. *Arterioscler Thromb* (1992) **12**:1063–70.

75 Rosendaal FR, Varekamp I, Smit C et al, Mortality and cause of death in Dutch haemophiliacs. 1973-86. *Br J Haematol* (1989) **71**:71–6.

76 Meade TW, Cooper JA, Stirling Y et al, Factor VIII, ABO blood group and the incidence of ischaemic heart disease. *Br J Haematol* (1994) **88**:601–7.

77 Thompson SG, Kienast J, Pyke SD, Hemostatic factors and the risk of myocardial infarction or sudden death in patients with angina pectoris. *N Engl J Med* (1995) **332**:635–41.

78 Ridker PM, Vaughan DE, Stampfer MJ, Endogenous tissue-type plasminogen activator and risk of myocardial infarction. *Lancet* (1993) **341**:1165–8.

79 Conlan MG. Folsom AR. Finch A. Davis CE et al, Associations of factor VIII and von Willebrand factor with age, sex and risk factors for atherosclerosis. *Thromb Haemost* (1993) **70**:380–5.

80 De Pergola G, De Mitrio V, Giorgino F et al, Increase in both pro-thrombotic and anti-thrombotic factors in obese premenopausal women: relationship with body fat distribution. *Int J Obesity* (1997) **21**:527–35.

81 Goldhaber SZ, Grodstein F, Stampfer MJ, Mason JE et al, A prospective study of risk factors for pulmonary embolism in women *JAMA* (1997) **277**:642–5.

82 Hannson PO, Eriksson H, Welin L, Svardsudd K, Wilhelmsen L, Smoking and abdominal obesity: risk factors for venous thromboembolism among middle-aged men: "the study of men born before 1913". *Arch Int Med* (1999) **159**:1886–90.

83 Kraaijenhagen RA, Anker PS, Koopman MM et al, High plasma concentration of factor VIIIc is a major risk factor for venous thromboembolism *Thromb Haemost* (2000) **83**:5–9.

84 Kyrle PA, Minar E, Hirschl M et al, High plasma levels of factor VIII and the risk of recurrent venous thromboembolism. *N Engl J Med* (2000) **343**:457–62.

85 Conlan MG, Folsom AR, Finch A et al, Correlation of plasma protein C levels with cardiovascular risk factors in middle-aged adults: the Atherosclerosis Risk in Communities (ARIC) Study. *Thromb Haemost* (1993) **70**:762–7.

Obesity and respiratory complications

Tracey D Robinson and Ronald R Grunstein

6

Introduction

Obesity can impact significantly on lung function, with excess central fat deposition producing a restrictive pulmonary abnormality and increased work of breathing. As a result, respiratory complaints are common in subjects with obesity and conditions such as asthma are often overdiagnosed in obese patients. Obesity is also strongly linked to breathing disorders during sleep, such as sleep apnoea and nocturnal hypoventilation. Sleep-disordered breathing has a number of clinical consequences, including impaired daytime gas exchange and excess cardiovascular morbidity. The combination of obesity-induced reduced pulmonary function and sleep-disordered breathing can lead to progressive respiratory failure during sleep, finally resulting in awake hypercapnic respiratory failure (obesity-hypoventilation syndrome, OHS). OHS can occur without any intrinsic lung disease. Weight reduction can improve lung function, reduce respiratory symptoms and reduce the severity of sleep apnoea. However, long-term maintenance of weight loss is difficult to achieve. Treatment of sleep-breathing disorders has been advanced greatly by the use of positive airway pressure devices and OHS can be reversed with the use of these devices.

Pulmonary function in obesity

Pulmonary function and mechanics in obesity

Lung volumes

Fat deposition in the neck, upper airway, chest wall and abdomen can impair the mechanical function of the respiratory system, usually by reducing lung volumes. In general, the effects of obesity alone are mild and are typically in proportion to the degree of obesity.[1–3] Falls in the expiratory reserve volume (ERV) and the functional residual capacity (FRC) are the commonest findings. Reductions in total lung capacity (TLC) and vital capacity (which would produce abnormal spirometry) are usually only seen in the morbidly obese, where the body mass index

(BMI) exceeds 40 kg/m². Even with obesity of this degree, the effects on TLC and VC are variable: measurements of central obesity correlate more closely with abnormalities of lung function than BMI.[4] Reductions in TLC and vital capacity to below 70% of predicted values are rarely due to obesity alone. Patients with OHS tend to have lower lung volumes than patients without sleep-disordered breathing, despite identical degrees of obesity (Table 6.1). The reasons for this are not clear, but may be related to the effects of chronic hypoventilation on lung compliance. After significant weight loss, either by caloric restriction or bariatric surgery, lung volumes increase towards normal.[5]

Lung mechanics

Obese subjects have an increased airway resistance compared to normal.[2] This increased resistance is largely due to the lower

Table 6.1
Representative lung volumes in two subjects with obesity and one patient with obesity-hypoventilation syndrome (OHS).

	FEV₁/FVC (ratio)	TLC (% predicted)	VC (% predicted)	FRC (% predicted)
Obese (BMI 35 kg/m²)	84	95	90	77
Obese (BMI 50 kg/m²)	83	86	79	75
OHS (BMI 48 kg/m²)	87	69	75	42

FEV_1/FVC = forced expiratory volume in one second/forced vital capacity; TLC = total lung capacity; VC = vital capacity; FRC = functional residual capacity; BMI = body mass index.

lung volumes seen in obesity resulting in a smaller airway calibre. Despite the increased resistance, the FEV_1/FVC ratio is usually normal.[1–3,6] Obese subjects also have 'stiffer' lungs than normals, with lung compliance reduced by around 25%. The reasons for this are unclear, but small airway closure and collapse may be responsible.

The fraction of total oxygen consumption dedicated to respiratory muscle work during quiet breathing can be up to 15% (that is, five times normal) in patients with morbid obesity, suggesting significantly increased work of breathing at rest. Respiratory muscle function as measured by maximal inspiratory and expiratory pressures is normal in eucapnic obese subjects, although respiratory muscle endurance may be reduced. In OHS, inspiratory muscles are weaker, possibly due to the effects of chronic hypoxaemia and hypercapnia.

Gas exchange in obesity

Hypoxaemia is seen in many patients with morbid obesity, but many patients with similar degrees of obesity have normal daytime gas exchange.[7,8] In obese hypoxaemic subjects, ventilation–perfusion mismatching has been demonstrated, with dependent well-perfused areas of lung relatively underventilated, probably due to partial airway collapse.[9] The gas exchange abnormalities are usually greater when patients are supine.

The presence of sleep-disordered breathing can impact significantly on waking gas exchange abnormalities and may explain some of the variation found in obese subjects. OHS describes the occurrence of hypercapnic hypoxaemic respiratory failure in obese patients who have no significant lung disease. The respiratory failure is largely due to impaired ventilatory control resulting in chronic awake alveolar hypoventilation. Patients with OHS can attain a normal $PaCO_2$ by voluntary hyperventilation.[10] However, the A–a PO_2 (alveolar–arterial oxygen gradient) is often increased in patients with OHS, suggesting the presence of increased ventilation–perfusion mismatch in addition to hypoventilation. The abnormal daytime ventilatory control is probably due to the combination of OSA and sleep-related hypoventilation causing profound nocturnal respiratory failure. The presence of OSA without OHS can also contribute to awake gas exchange abnormalities. Laaban et al[11] studied a group of 60 obese subjects (BMI around 50 kg/m^2) and found that daytime hypoxaemia was significantly correlated with the presence of OSA. Similar findings have been reported by Gold et al.[8] This mild to moderate hypoxaemia with eucapnia seen in obese patients with OSA is probably attributable to abnormalities of ventilatory control causing mild hypoventilation: this group may represent an early form of OHS.

The single-breath diffusing capacity for

carbon monoxide (DLCO), a measure of the gas exchange capacity of the lung, is increased in obese subjects by about 10%. When DLCO is corrected for lung volume (KCO), increases of around 25% are seen in obese subjects.[12] The cause is unclear, but may be related to increased pulmonary capillary blood volume.

Control of breathing in obesity

Ventilatory control is usually assessed by measuring responses to chemical stimuli such as hypercapnia and hypoxaemia. There is a wide variation in normal responses to these tests. In patients with uncomplicated obesity, ventilatory drive is usually normal. Reduced ventilatory responses to hypercapnia have been reported in obese patients with OSA.[8] By definition, patients with OHS (daytime alveolar hypoventilation) have impaired ventilatory control and these patients can often voluntarily hyperventilate their $PaCO_2$ down to normal levels. On formal testing, patients with OHS often have blunted ventilatory responses to hypoxia and hypercapnia, although typically there is a shift in CO_2 responsiveness, characterized by a normal slope of the ventilatory response to CO_2, albeit at a higher level of $PaCO_2$.[13] Both familial factors and lifetime alcohol intake can influence ventilatory drive, possibly predisposing obese subjects to the development of OHS. However, a role for OSA and sleep-disordered breathing in the genesis of OHS is strongly suggested by studies demonstrating improvements in ventilatory responses after a period of treatment of OSA with CPAP.

Respiratory symptoms in obesity

Does obesity alone, in the absence of cardiorespiratory disease, cause exertional breathlessness, wheeze and chest discomfort? The Swedish Obese Subjects Study (SOS) reported an increased incidence of respiratory symptoms, in particular exertional breathlessness and chest discomfort in obese, otherwise healthy subjects compared to normal weight subjects.[14] Interestingly, when subjects with similar degrees of obesity were compared, those patients with OSA reported more exertional dyspnoea than those without OSA.[15] There was a significant reduction in these symptoms with weight loss following bariatric surgery,[16] with an independent association between the reduction in sleep-disordered breathing and the relief of breathlessness and chest pain. This suggests that sleep-disordered breathing has a role in the genesis of these symptoms in subjects with obesity, possibly through impaired respiratory control and mild daytime hypoxaemia. In the absence of weight loss, CPAP therapy can improve daytime gas exchange and respiratory control in patients with obesity and OSA,[17] and so may relieve daytime respiratory symptoms in obese subjects with OSA.

Obesity is significantly associated with an increased incidence of gastro-oesophageal reflux disease. Reflux is a common cause of chronic persistent cough and cough may be the only symptom of reflux disease.

Obesity and asthma

Is obesity an independent risk factor for asthma? A number of recent studies have described an epidemiological association between obesity and asthma.[18] However, the diagnosis of asthma in these studies was not confirmed with tests of bronchial hyper-responsiveness (BHR) such as bronchoprovocation challenge or 24 hour peak flow variability. In the absence of such testing, the false-positive diagnosis rate for asthma can be as high as 65%. A more recent study showed an increased incidence of doctor-diagnosed asthma and asthma medication usage in obese subjects but found no increase in the incidence of BHR or atopy in obese subjects compared to normals.[19] This suggests that asthma is overdiagnosed and overtreated in obese subjects, possibly due to the respiratory symptoms associated with obesity alone. Weight loss, either by dietary means or by bariatric surgery, can result in a reduction in asthma symptoms and medication usage.[20,21] However, these studies did not demonstrate changes in BHR. This

suggests that the reduction in respiratory symptoms is due to the reduction in weight and improvement in obesity-associated conditions such as sleep disordered breathing or gastro-oesophageal reflux, rather than to a change in the severity of asthma.

Sleep-disordered breathing: background

Background

Sleep physiologists consider humans to exist in three states – wakefulness, nonrapid eye movement (NREM) sleep and rapid eye movement (REM or dreaming) sleep, with marked physiological changes between these states. During sleep in normal subjects, there are falls in minute ventilation, pharyngeal muscle tone and chemosensitivity to chemical stimuli (for example hypoxia or hypercapnia). Furthermore, in REM sleep breathing irregularity occurs and postural muscle tone is lost. This means we depend solely on the diaphragm for breathing during REM sleep. Any patient with abnormal respiratory function when awake will have significantly impaired breathing and gas exchange when asleep, particularly during REM sleep.

Definitions

Sleep-disordered breathing describes a range of conditions from simple snoring through to profound nocturnal hypoventilation and respiratory failure. Obstructive sleep apnoea (OSA) is characterized by repetitive episodes of reduction in or complete cessation of airflow during sleep secondary to complete or partial collapse of the pharyngeal airway (Figure 6.1). During an obstructive apnoea, continued respiratory efforts occur against the collapsed airway, typically leading to hypoxaemia (which can be profound) until the apnoea is terminated by arousal and upper airway patency is re-established. After a few deep breaths (often loud snores), this cycle is repeated as often as 200–600 times per night. The recurrent arousals result in dramatically fragmented sleep, with loss of normal sleep architecture leading to severe sleepiness during the day.

Clinically significant upper airway obstruction may occur in the absence of complete collapse of the upper airway. Partial obstruction (hypopnoea) may produce similar pathophysiological events (that is, hypoxaemia and arousal). Even minor increases in airway resistance can be associated with repetitive arousal and excessive daytime sleepiness; the 'upper airway resistance' syndrome.[22]

Pathogenesis of sleep apnoea

Collapse of the upper airway occurs when the negative (or suction) pressure applied to the upper airway during inspiration is greater than the dilating force applied by upper airway muscles, such as genioglossus.[23] Any factors which reduce airway size, decrease muscle

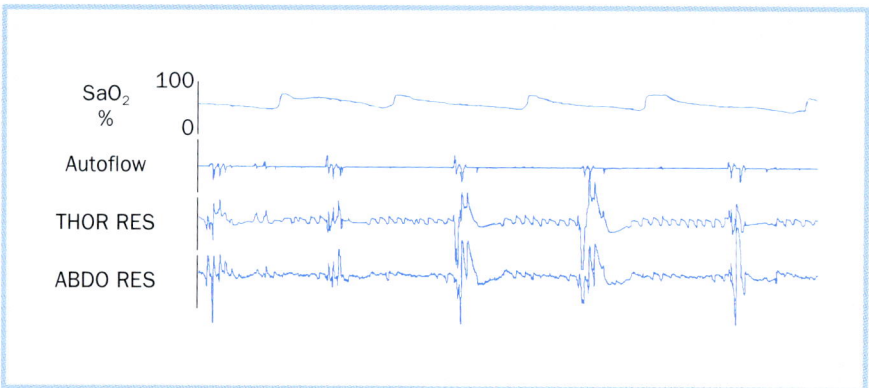

Figure 6.1
Five-minute tracing of a patient with typical severe sleep apnoea. The apnoeas are indicated by intermittent cessation of airflow (Autoflow: nasal airflow) and are obstructive in nature, as continued respiratory effort is seen when airflow is absent (THOR RES: thoracic movement or effort; ABDO RES: abdominal movement or effort). Repetitive falls in oxygen saturation (SaO_2) are seen following each apnoea.

tone, increase upper airway compliance or lead to generation of a greater inspiratory pressure will predispose to OSA. Muscle tone and suction pressure are influenced by sleep stage and relative respiratory drive to the diaphragm versus the upper airway dilator muscles.

In general, obese patients with OSA have larger tongues and smaller upper airways than normal subjects. In morbidly obese patients, neck size is a better predictor of sleep apnoea than other body anthropomorphic measures:[15] presumably neck fat deposition promotes mass loading and obstruction of the upper airway in sleep, leading to OSA. However, in a wider weight range of patients with OSA, waist circumference was a better predictor of OSA than neck circumference,[24] and excess fat deposition around the airway is not a universal finding in obese patients with OSA. There is some evidence for a functional abnormality in upper airway muscles in obese subjects, possibly due to fat deposition. Abdominal obesity can reduce lung volumes, leading to a reduction in pharyngeal cross-sectional area and increased pharyngeal resistance. Obesity may promote sleep apnoea through multiple mechanisms: in some patients, neck fat deposition may be the critical factor causing upper airway closure in sleep; in other patients, abdominal fat loading may be important.

Obesity-hypoventilation syndrome

Most patients with OSA have normal arterial carbon dioxide tensions when awake. The association between obesity, hypersomnolence and daytime respiratory failure (the obesity-hypoventilation syndrome, Pickwickian syndrome) has been reported for many years, but the pathogenesis was poorly understood. The recognition that sleep apnoea was present in these patients and that relief of upper airway obstruction by tracheostomy effectively treated the respiratory failure altered the understanding of the evolution of OHS. Upper airway obstruction is a crucial factor in the pathogenesis of OHS.[23] However, since most OSA patients do not have hypercapnia when awake, upper airway obstruction alone is insufficient to cause OHS. Similarly, obesity, per se, is associated with normal chemosensitivity.

There are no longitudinal studies on the development of OHS, but sleep-induced respiratory abnormalities almost certainly occur before the development of daytime respiratory failure. During an apnoea, $PaCO_2$ rises and PaO_2 falls. When the apnoea is terminated by arousal, ventilation increases and oxygen and carbon dioxide levels can return to normal. If arousal responses or ventilatory responses to either hypoxia or hypercapnia are depressed, the apnoeic periods will be longer, the degree of blood gas derangement greater and normalization of blood gases in the period following arousal compromised.[23] In those patients able to increase ventilation between apnoeas, overall eucapnia will be maintained. If the compensatory mechanisms are poor, persistent hypercapnia and hypoxia will occur during sleep. This will eventually allow the resetting of chemoreceptors,[13] tolerance of higher waking CO_2 levels and progression to daytime hypercapnia. Family studies suggest that ventilatory responses to hypercapnia and hypoxia are influenced by genetic factors. Arousal responses may be further impaired in patients prescribed sedatives/hypnotics to improve 'insomnia' or by consumption of alcohol. Lifetime heavy alcohol intake may also impair ventilatory responses.

It is likely that the key elements in the development of OHS are a combination of obesity (increased upper airway loading and reduced lung volumes), OSA, poor chemoreceptor function (particularly defective arousal responses to hypoxia) and possibly alcohol consumption (reducing upper airway

tone and arousal responses to asphyxia).[23] It is important to stress that awake hypercapnia can occur in obese patients in the absence of any smoking history or lung disease.[25] The prevalence of OHS in the obese population is unknown, but it is probably underdiagnosed. A recent study found that 31% of obese patients (BMI > 35 kg/m^2) admitted to medical wards had OHS.[26]

Sleep-disordered breathing: epidemiology

The general community

Daytime sleepiness and snoring are commonly reported symptoms in the general community, and sleepiness may have many causes (Table 6.2). Snoring may be underestimated if history from a bed partner is unavailable. Questionnaire estimates of OSA are therefore difficult to interpret.

The Wisconsin Sleep Cohort study[27] is the largest reported prevalence study where sleep

Table 6.2
Causes of sleepiness in the obese patient.

Not enough sleep	Lifestyle, insomnia
Drugs causing sleepiness	Hypnotics, drug abuse
Sleep-disrupting disorders	OSA, PLMS
Primary brain disorders	Narcolepsy, IHS

OSA: obstructive sleep apnoea; PLMS: periodic limb movement disorder; IHS: idiopathic hypersomnolence.

studies were performed. This group found an apnoea index of >5 events per hour in 9% of female and 24% of male middle-aged public servants. The 'OSA syndrome' (daytime sleepiness and an apnoea index of >5 per hour) was found in 2% of women and 4% of men. An apnoea index of >15 per hour (a criterion which would satisfy most sleep researchers) was found in 4% of women and 9% of men with sleep apnoea. Our group has found a similar prevalence of OSA in an Australian rural community using home monitoring of breathing.[28]

The obese population

Studies have consistently shown that obesity, especially central obesity, is strongly associated with sleep-disordered breathing in adults.[24,27,28] Measurements of central obesity such as waist or neck circumferences are tightly linked to OSA in sleep clinic populations.[24] In the Busselton Sleep Survey,[28] there was a powerful effect of BMI in increasing the risk of SDB in the community (Figure 6.2). There are limited data on the prevalence of sleep apnoea in the obese population. Data from the Swedish Obese Subjects (SOS) study, which examined 3034

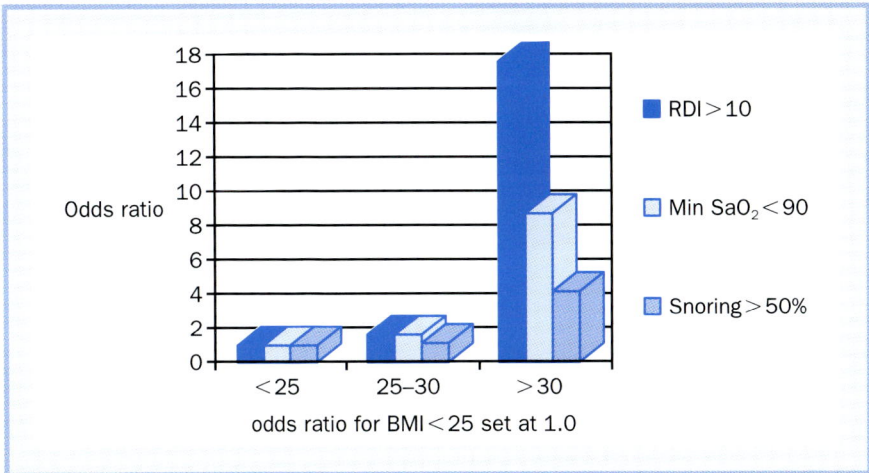

Figure 6.2
Obesity (measured by BMI) is an important predictor of OSA. With the odds ratio for BMI < 25 set at 1.0, a BMI > 30 increased the odds ratio of either OSA (respiratory disturbance index RDI > 10), desaturation during the night (min SaO_2 < 90%) or heavy snoring (snoring for more than 50% of the night) by 5–18 times, depending on the variable.

subjects with BMI >35 kg/m², found that over 50% of obese men and one-third of obese women reported habitual loud snoring.[15] In the SOS study, a history of frequent witnessed apnoeas (a sensitive marker of sleep apnoea in epidemiological studies) was reported by 33% of men and 12% of women. The exact prevalence of the spectrum of sleep-breathing disorders in the obese is unknown, but it is clear that OSA and related conditions occur in a very high proportion of obese subjects.

Other risk factors for sleep apnoea

OSA increases in prevalence with age and is commonly recognized in the fifth and seventh decades. Some of the increase in prevalence with age is due to increased central fat deposition with age. The male to female ratio in sleep apnoea is close to 2.5:1.[27,28] Sleep apnoea is rare in premenopausal women unless there is morbid obesity or maxillo-facial abnormalities. The prevalence of OSA increases in women after the menopause, suggesting that female sex hormones are protective or male hormones may promote OSA. Alternatively, the increased prevalence in OSA after the menopause may be secondary to changing body fat distribution in postmenopausal women.

Apart from upper airway fat secondary to obesity, other conditions causing narrowing of the upper airway will promote the development of sleep apnoea. These include fixed upper airway lesions such as nasal obstruction and enlarged tonsils, macroglossia and neurological conditions impairing upper airway muscle tone. Sleep apnoea aggregates in families and the risk of having OSA increases progressively with increasing numbers of affected relatives. This may be the result of similarities in facial structure affecting upper airway dynamics in sleep. Certain maxillo-facial appearances are linked with sleep apnoea. In obese patients, familial maxillo-mandibular structure will interact to increase the likelihood of sleep apnoea. This may explain why weight loss may not be enough to cure sleep apnoea in obese patients.[29]

A number of endocrine and metabolic disorders apart from obesity are associated with an increased prevalence of OSA. Hypothyroidism can lead to sleep apnoea by reducing chemosensitivity, causing airway narrowing due to myxoedematous infiltration and upper airway myopathy. Over 50% of patients with acromegaly have sleep apnoea.[30] Cushing's disease is also associated with sleep apnoea.

Acute alcohol ingestion promotes apnoea development during later sleep. Lifetime alcohol consumption may be a risk factor for the development of OSA. Data from the Wisconsin Sleep Cohort suggest that smoking history may be a dose-dependent risk factor for OSA.

Cardiac failure (whatever the cause) is associated with a high incidence of sleep-disordered breathing. In a recent study of 450 patients with cardiac failure referred to a sleep laboratory (either with sleep symptoms or persistent dyspnoea), 72% had more than 10 apnoeas–hypopnoeas per hour.[31] Patients had OSA or central sleep apnoea (Cheynes–Stokes respiration), with OSA more common in those patients with BMI > 35 kg/m².

Sleep-disordered breathing: clinical

Symptoms and signs

History and physical examination have surprisingly poor sensitivity and specificity for the detection of sleep-disordered breathing. The classic symptoms associated with OSA are heavy snoring and excessive daytime sleepiness (EDS). The occurrence of witnessed apnoeas is a relatively specific symptom, but is also relatively insensitive. Other symptoms are listed in Table 6.3. Daytime symptoms include morning headaches, fatigue, poor memory and concentration, alteration in mood and impotence.

The nature of these symptoms emphasizes the importance of obtaining a history from the spouse, bed partner or other family members. Few patients are aware that they snore or stop breathing during sleep. Excessive sleepiness may be recognized by the patient,

Table 6.3
Symptoms of sleep-disordered breathing.

Snoring
Choking in sleep
Disrupted sleep at night
Daytime sleepiness
Dry throat
Palpitations in sleep
Nocturia
Heartburn
Headaches (day or night)
Fatigue
Poor memory and concentration
Alteration in mood, irritability
Impotence

but is often under-reported as patients are either unaware that their sleepiness is abnormal or fearful of potential consequences (such as loss of driving licence or work).

Examination of the upper airway may be important. Obvious pharyngeal crowding and tonsillar enlargement suggest upper airway obstruction. The vibration associated with heavy snoring can lead to a reddened and oedematous uvula and soft palate. Systemic hypertension is commonly associated with OSA.

Diagnosis

An overnight sleep study (polysomnography) is the 'gold standard' for the investigation of sleep-disordered breathing. During a full sleep study, sleep stage is monitored along with measures of airflow at the nose/mouth, measures of respiratory effort, such as diaphragm EMG and chest wall and abdominal movement, and other important variables including oxygen saturation, ECG and leg EMG. The sleep study report should include the total amount of sleep and proportions of different sleep stages, the number of respiratory events seen (apnoeas and hypopnoeas per hour both in REM and nonREM sleep), the degree of oxygen desaturation recorded, the number of EEG arousals and the presence or absence of periodic leg movements. Definitions of events are not standard in all sleep laboratories and different methods for measuring respiratory variables have differing sensitivities, particularly in the measurement of airflow.

In general, an apnoea–hypopnoea index (AHI) of less than 5 events per hour would be considered normal, with an AHI of greater than 15 events per hour considered significant. The clinical importance of an index of 5 to 15 events per hour is uncertain, particularly in the elderly, but there is significant individual variability in this area. If a patient is symptomatic, then a trial of treatment is warranted. More recent studies have suggested that an AHI as low as 5 may significantly increase the risk of developing hypertension.[32]

There can be significant night-to-night variability in the severity of sleep-disordered breathing, and potential causes for a false-negative sleep study are listed in Table 6.4. A negative study with high clinical suspicion warrants further review and perhaps even a repeat sleep study.

The expense and inconvenience of polysomnography has led to a search for alternative tools for the diagnosis of OSA. Overnight oximetry can detect repetitive oxygen desaturations seen in OSA (Figure 6.3) and may be diagnostic in some patients. However, events not associated with significant desaturation will be missed and so this test does not exclude OSA. Similarly, limited and portable or 'at-home' systems have been used with some success in the diagnosis of OSA, but again do not exclude the diagnosis if negative. They are probably most useful in those patients who cannot readily be studied in a laboratory and where the clinical suspicion is high.

Table 6.4
Reasons for false-negative sleep studies.

Poor sleep efficiency (laboratory effect)
Little or no REM sleep seen
Usual sedatives or alcohol not taken
Patient not sleeping in usual position (especially supine)
Occurrence of 'subcriterion events'
Night-to-night variability in OSA (significant in milder disease)

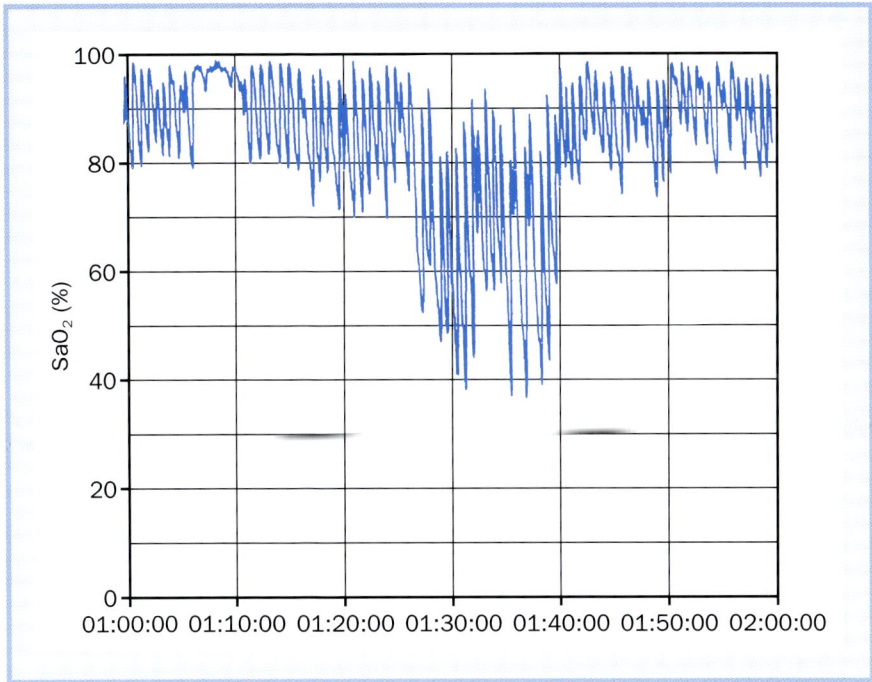

Figure 6.3
One-hour oximetry recording during sleep in a patient with OSA, showing typical repetitive arterial oxygen desaturations. The greatest desaturations occur from 01:25 to 01:40 hours, when the patient is in REM sleep.

Consequences

Psychosocial

Excessive daytime sleepiness (EDS) is characteristic but not pathognomonic of sleep apnoea. Sleepiness in OSA is predominantly related to the repetitive arousals with subsequent sleep fragmentation, but a direct

effect of hypoxaemia is possible. There is a relatively poor correlation between markers of severity of OSA, such as AHI, and daytime sleepiness and no simple test accurately quantifies daytime sleepiness. Sleepiness can lead both to impaired work performance and impaired driving. It is clear that sleepy patients with OSA form an important risk group for motor vehicle accidents. Treatment with nasal CPAP dramatically improves daytime sleepiness, quality of life and even driving simulator performance. A number of studies have found OSA patients perform poorly on psychometric tests compared to controls, with a variable degree of improvement following nasal CPAP therapy.[33] Data from the Swedish Obese Subjects study indicate that in equally obese men and women, a history of sleep apnoea is associated with impaired work performance, increased sick leave and a much higher divorce rate.

Cardiovascular

Patients with sleep apnoea clearly have a number of acute cardiovascular changes as an immediate consequence of their breathing disturbance. Obstructive apnoeas are accompanied by profound haemodynamic changes, with increases in both systemic and pulmonary arterial blood pressure. With progressive apnoea, there is worsening hypoxaemia, increasing pleural pressure swings, bradycardia (and possibly bradyarrhythmias), increased sympathetic nerve activity and an overall rise in blood pressure. These marked changes in cardiorespiratory function, together with reported changes in cerebral blood flow, provide an environment for increasing the risk of vascular disease endpoints. Studies using a canine model of OSA have shown that

sustained hypertension develops after 1 to 3 months of OSA.[34] Similarly, studies with rats have found that intermittent hypoxia induces a persistent increase in diurnal blood pressure, possibly mediated through renal sympathetic nerve activity and the renin–angiotensin system.[35]

Sleep apnoea is a common finding in hypertension clinic patients, but there are confounding factors such as central obesity and increasing age.[24] A number of studies have strongly suggested that sleep apnoea is a risk factor for hypertension independent of obesity.[15,24] Recently published cross-sectional data from the Sleep Heart Health study show a significant association between sleep-disordered breathing and hypertension after adjustment for BMI, neck circumference and waist to hip ratio.[36] Similarly, prospective data from the Wisconsin Sleep Cohort study have found a dose–response association between sleep-disordered breathing and hypertension, independent of measures of obesity.[32] Studies using either intrarterial monitoring, automated daytime blood pressure readings or 24-hour ambulatory blood pressure have demonstrated a fall in blood pressure levels after CPAP treatment.

Patients with OSA have increased left ventricular mass (measured using echocardiography) compared with nonOSA patients with similar daytime blood pressure values. A number of groups have reported an increased risk of myocardial infarction and stroke in sleep apnoea.[37] Snoring is a strong risk factor for sleep-related strokes, while sleep apnoea symptoms (snoring plus reported apnoeas or EDS) increase the risk of cerebral infarction, with an odds ratio of 8.0. Pulmonary hypertension can develop as a consequence of OSA alone.[38] These observations in OSA have implications in the analysis of data linking obesity and cardiac disease.

The advent of nasal CPAP has prevented large studies investigating the natural history of untreated OSA. He et al observed an increased cumulative mortality in untreated patients with an apnoea index (AI) > 20 compared to AI < 20.[39] Tracheostomy or CPAP treatment, but not uvulopalatopharyngoplasty (UPPP), reduced the mortality risk. More recently, untreated OSA has been found to be associated with an increased cardiovascular mortality in patients with coronary artery disease.

Endocrine

Sleep apnoea patients have a neuroendocrine defect in both growth hormone (GH) and testosterone secretion. This abnormality can be reversed by nasal CPAP treatment without associated weight change. In adults, impaired GH secretion leads to central adiposity and reduced muscle and bone mass, but it is unknown whether these changes in GH and testosterone levels in adults with sleep apnoea

are associated with measurable changes in body composition, body fat distribution, energy expenditure or bone density. Reports have suggested that insulin levels are increased in patients with sleep apnoea independent of obesity or visceral fat mass.[15] Other data strongly suggest that reversal of sleep apnoea leads to increased insulin sensitivity in obese type 2 diabetic patients and to reduced visceral fat mass.[40] More recently, leptin has been implicated in sleep-disordered breathing. In obese, leptin-deficient mice with OHS, leptin replacement increased both waking and sleeping minute ventilation and chemosensitivity to carbon dioxide during sleep.[41] Patients with OSA have higher leptin levels than subjects with similar obesity without OSA. Leptin levels fell significantly in a group of 22 patients with OSA after 4 days of treatment with CPAP,[40] possibly due to reduced sympathetic activity. OSA may well be a confounder in some of the hormonal associations observed in central obesity and is possibly associated with leptin resistance.

Treatment of sleep apnoea and snoring

The approach to treatment should be determined by the severity of symptoms, the severity of hypoxaemia during sleep and possibly by the presence of associated cardiovascular risk factors, although this is a difficult and controversial area. Patient occupation may also influence treatment decisions. Importantly, patient denial may produce an 'asymptomatic' patient – always check with family if there is a highly positive study in an asymptomatic patient.

Weight loss and lifestyle factors

Weight loss, either through dietary means or by bariatric surgery will significantly reduce the severity of OSA, but the effect is variable and therefore it is important to re-assess patients after weight loss. Recent data from the Swedish Obese Subjects study have shown a marked reduction in sleep apnoea symptomatology in obese subjects 2 years after surgically-induced weight loss compared with controls. However, complete cure of all sleep-disordered breathing with weight loss is rare: many patients have significant residual disease that warrants further treatment.[42]

Reduction of smoking and alcohol consumption can lead to reduced self-reported snoring and reverse mild sleep apnoea. Sleep deprivation can reduce upper airway tone and chemosensitivity and should be avoided in patients with OSA. Similarly, drugs such as benzodiazepines or opiates should be avoided at bedtime.

Devices

Positive airway pressure

Prior to the advent of nasal continuous positive airway pressure (CPAP) in 1981, tracheostomy was the only form of treatment available for sleep apnoea and was usually only performed in patients with severe symptomatic disease. Nasal CPAP has revolutionized the field of sleep-disordered breathing and is the most effective treatment available for OSA.[43,44] A CPAP machine delivers varying pressure to the upper airway through a nose or face mask, providing a 'pneumatic' splint which prevents upper airway closure (Figure 6.4). CPAP treatment leads to normalization of sleep architecture, decreased upper airway oedema and a reduction in daytime sleepiness.[44,45] CPAP improves cognitive function, mood and quality of life, as well as the associated symptoms listed in Table 6.1 for patients with all degrees of severity of OSA.[46] Evidence also suggests that CPAP reduces the incidence of actual and near-miss car accidents. CPAP is not a cure for sleep apnoea. Cessation of treatment will lead to a recurrence of sleep-disordered breathing and accompanying symptoms.

Compliance is the main problem with CPAP. Various studies report compliance ranging from 40 to 80%. The machine and mask remain cumbersome and inconvenient. Side effects of treatment are common and,

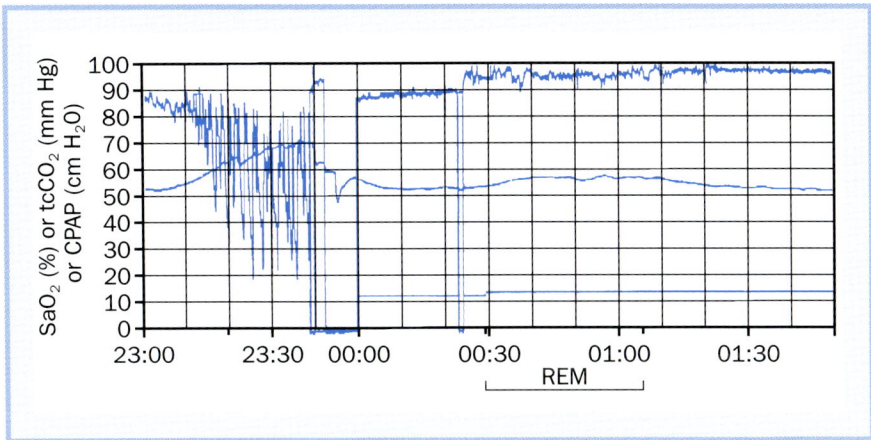

Figure 6.4
Two-hour oximetry recording, with transcutaneous (tc) CO_2 monitoring in a patient with severe OSA during a split-night study (part-diagnostic, part-treatment). From 23:00 to 23:40 hours, the patient is in diagnostic mode, with repetitive arterial oxygen desaturations and rising $tcCO_2$. From 00:00 onwards, the patient is on nasal CPAP with maintenance of arterial oxygen saturation above 90% and prevention of rises in $tcCO_2$.

although minor, may reduce compliance. Poorly fitting masks can cause skin irritation and even ulceration. Nasal congestion, rhinitis, epistaxis and dryness of the mouth and throat can occur and are usually associated with mask or mouth airleaks. Humidification of the inspired air can reduce some of these problems, as can careful attention to mask fit. Education and early follow-up may improve compliance. Patients with mild disease or those requiring high pressures are most likely to be noncompliant. Obese patients generally require higher CPAP pressures.

Newer devices that allow differing inspiratory and expiratory pressures (triggered by the patient's respiratory cycle) are known as bi-level positive airway pressure machines and were originally introduced to improve compliance in CPAP users. Although not proven to improve compliance, this form of positive airway pressure therapy, which essentially provides pressure support ventilation, has been used increasingly in the management of severe respiratory failure and hypoventilation during sleep, such as OHS.

Mandibular advancement splints

Mandibular advancement splints are orthodontic devices designed to displace the mandible anteriorly, increasing the anteroposterior diameter of the upper airway and so potentially reducing collapse when worn at night. Several studies have shown a significant reduction in sleep apnoea severity with these devices. These devices require careful orthodontic attention to ensure that adequate anterior displacement of the mandible is achieved. The efficacy of these devices is likely to be reduced in the obese patient as skeletal factors and maxillo-facial abnormalities are less important in the genesis of upper airway obstruction. In general, these devices tend to be less effective in those patients with severe OSA,[47] and few data are available on compliance and the prevalence of side effects related to the temporomandibular joint.

Surgery

Tracheostomy

Before the availability of nasal CPAP, tracheostomy was the only effective therapeutic modality for OSA. It is an extremely invasive procedure, associated with significant morbidity, particularly in the obese fat-necked individual, and is only partially effective in treating OHS. Tracheostomy is only indicated in those patients with severe OSA who are unable to tolerate CPAP or other therapy. Prior to consideration of surgery, the patient should be fully reviewed,

with intensive attempts to introduce CPAP. Some patients may warrant ENT review/intervention to facilitate CPAP usage. With skilful surgery and close follow-up, tracheostomy may be a 'last-resort' therapeutic option in some patients.

Uvulopalatopharyngoplasty and other upper airway surgery

Uvulopalatopharyngoplasty (UPPP) involves careful removal of the uvula and part of the soft palate and was originally intended to treat heavy snoring. The efficacy of UPPP in the treatment of OSA is limited. When treatment success is defined as a reduction in AHI of only 50%, a successful result is seen in only 50% of patients. There are no pre-operative tests that satisfactorily predict the response to surgery. There is a significant morbidity and even mortality. Excessive removal of palatal tissue can lead to velo-pharyngeal incompetence with nasal regurgitation and speech changes. Subsequent use of CPAP may be more difficult following UPPP. Many studies report particularly poor results in obese patients.

More recently UPPP has been performed with a surgical laser or high-frequency radio waves ('somnoplasty'), aiming at stiffening palatal tissue rather than removal. The treatment response is variable and unpredictable, with a poor relationship between subjective and objective measures of efficacy.[48] There is clearly a 'placebo' effect in snoring surgery that has been demonstrated in other forms of surgical intervention.

More complex maxillo-facial surgery, usually involving UPPP in combination with genioglossus advancement via a mandibular osteotomy and hyoid myotomy, has been used with some success in the treatment of OSA. However, this surgery is less effective in patients with severe disease (>60 events per hour and desaturation to 70%) and in the morbidly obese.[49] These complex surgical procedures are not widely available.

Management of sleep apnoea with awake respiratory failure including OHS

Depending on the chronicity and the severity of the respiratory failure, these patients are often best managed during a brief hospital admission. While most patients starting CPAP require only one night of sleep monitoring to determine required pressure adequately, patients with sleep apnoea and awake respiratory failure require more detailed assessment. In these patients, oxygen alone should be used with caution and with close monitoring of hypercapnia, and sedation or use of hypnotics is contraindicated. Until recently, high CPAP pressures or CPAP plus added oxygen were needed in the first weeks of treatment until blood gases improved. However the newer bi-level positive airway pressure systems can deliver effective noninvasive pressure support ventilation to these patients and successfully treat hypercapnic respiratory failure (Figure 6.5). Home use of these devices is then prescribed with or without oxygen, depending on the degree of intrinsic lung disease. These patients are best managed by a specialist sleep unit with expertise in the management of sleep-related respiratory failure.

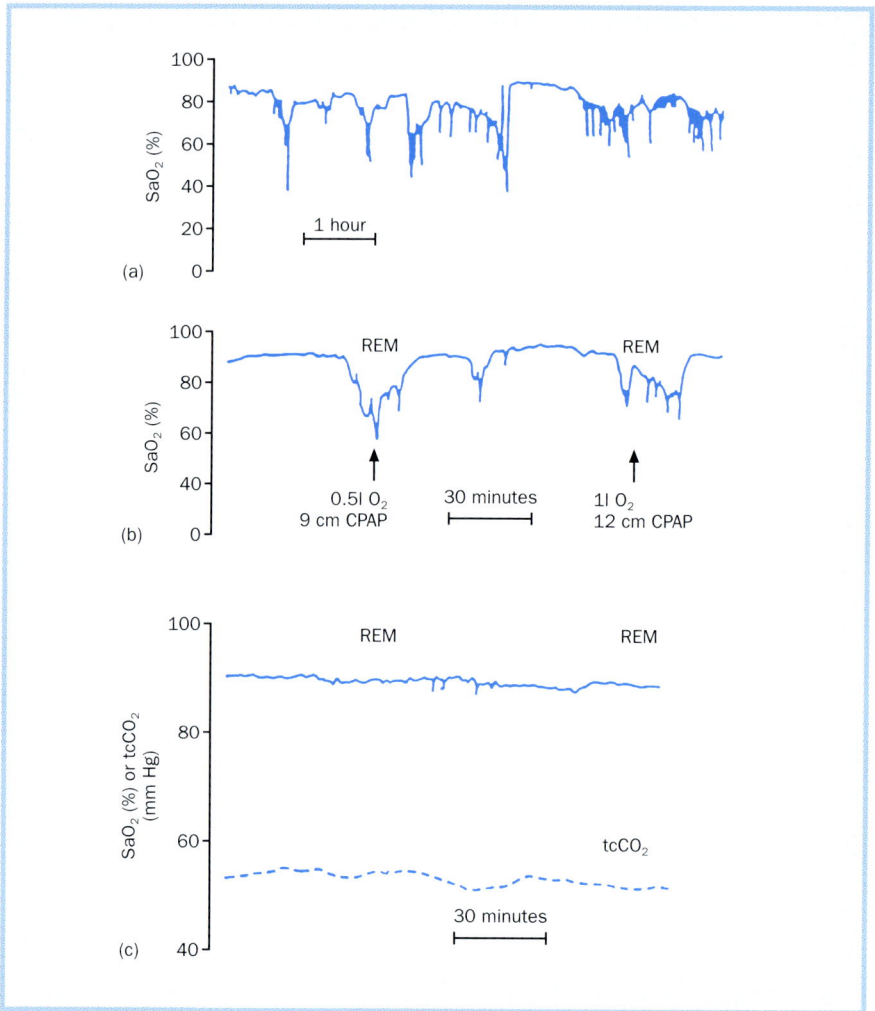

Figure 6.5
Efficacy of nasal ventilation in a patient with OHS. Recordings of oxygen saturation (SaO$_2$, %) show marked falls in oxygen level during sleep (a). Addition of CPAP and low-flow oxygen (0.5 l = 0.5 l/minute of supplemental oxygen; 1 l = 1 l/minute) results in normal oxygen saturation in NREM sleep but persisting hypoxaemia in REM sleep (b). Use of nasal ventilation, either pressure support or volume cycled, will prevent oxygen desaturation in REM sleep (c) and prevent rises in transcutaneous CO$_2$ (tcCO$_2$) levels.

References

1 Ray CS, Sue DY, Bray G et al, Effects of obesity on respiratory function, *Am Rev Resp Dis* (1983) **128**:501–6.

2 Zerah F, Harf A, Perlemuter L et al, Effects of obesity on respiratory resistance, *Chest* (1993) **103**:1470–6.

3 Jenkins SC, Moxham J, The effects of mild obesity on lung function, *Resp Med* (1991) **85**:309–11.

4 Collins LC, Hoberty PD, Walker JF et al, The effect of body fat distribution on pulmonary function tests, *Chest* (1995) **107**:1298–302.

5 Weiner P, Waizman J, Weiner M et al, Influence of excessive weight loss after gastroplasty for morbid obesity on respiratory muscle performance, *Thorax* (1998) **53**:39–42.

6 Lopata M, Onal E, Mass loading, sleep apnea, and the pathogenesis of obesity hypoventilation, *Am Rev Resp Dis* (1982) **126**:640–5.

7 Barrera F, Hillyer P, Ascanio G, Bechteh J, The distribution of ventilation, diffusion and blood flow in obese patients with normal and abnormal blood gases, *Am Rev Resp Dis* (1973) **108**:819–30.

8 Gold AR, Schwartz AR, Wise RA, Smith PL, Pulmonary function and respiratory chemosensitivity in moderately obese patients with sleep apnoea, *Chest* (1993) **103**:1325–9.

9 Barrera F, Reidenberg MM, Winters WL, Hungspreugs S, Ventilation–perfusion relationship in the obese patient, *J Appl Physiol* (1969) **26**:420–6.

10 Leech J, Onal E, Aronson R, Lopata M, Voluntary hyperventilation in obesity hypoventilation, *Chest* (1991) **100**:1334–8.

11 Laaban JP, Cassuto D, Orvoen-Frija E et al, Cardiorespiratory consequences of sleep apnoea syndrome in patients with massive obesity, *Eur Resp J* (1997) **11**:20–7.

12 Collard P, Wilputte J, Aubert G et al, The single-breath diffusing capacity for carbon monoxide in obstructive sleep apnoea and obesity, *Chest* (1996) **110**:1189–93.

13 Berthon-Jones M, Sullivan CE, Time course of change in ventilatory response to CO_2 with long-term CPAP therapy for obstructive sleep apnea, *Am Rev Resp Dis* (1987) **35**:144–7.

14 Sjostrom L, Larsson B, Backman L et al, Swedish Obese Subjects (SOS): recruitment for an intervention study and a selected description of the obese state, *Int J Obes Relat Metab Disord* (1992) **16**:465–79.

15 Grunstein RR, Stenlöf K, Hedner JA, Sjostrom L, Impact of sleep apnea and sleepiness on metabolic and cardiovascular risk factors in the Swedish Obese Subjects (SOS) Study, *Int J Obes Relat Metab Disord* (1995) **19**:410–18.

16 Karason K, Lindross AK, Stenlöf K, Sjostrom L, Relief of cardiorespiratory symptoms and increased physical activity after surgically induced weight loss, *Arch Intern Med* (2000) **160**:1797–802.

17 Sforza E, Krieger J, Wietzenblum E et al, Long-term effects of treatment with nasal continuous positive airway pressure on daytime lung function and pulmonary haemodynamics in patients with obstructive sleep apnoea, *Am Rev Resp Dis* (1990) **141**:866–70.

18 Camargo CA, Weiss ST, Zhang S et al, Prospective study of body mass index, weight change and risk of adult-onset asthma in women, *Arch Intern Med* (1999) **159**:2582–8.

19 Schachter LM, Salome CM, Peat JK, Woolcock AJ, Obesity is a risk factor for asthma and wheeze but not for airway hyperresponsiveness, *Thorax* (2000) **56**:4–8.

20 Dixon JB, Chapman L, O'Brien P, Marked improvement in asthma after lap-band surgery for morbid obesity, *Obes Surg* (1999) **9**:385–9.

21 Stenius-Aarniala B, Poussa T, Kvarnstrom J et al, Immediate and long term effects of weight reduction in obese people with asthma: randomised controlled study, *Br Med J* (2000) **320**:827–32.

22 Guilleminault C, Stoohs R, Clerk A et al, From obstructive sleep apnea syndrome to upper airway resistance syndrome: consistency of daytime sleepiness, *Sleep* (1992) **15**:513–16.

23 Sullivan CE, Grunstein RR, Marrone O, Berthon-Jones M, Sleep apnea – pathophysiology: upper airway and control of breathing. In: Guilleminault C, Partinnen M, eds, *Obstructive Sleep Apnea Syndrome: Clinical Research and Treatment* (Raven Press: New York, 1990).

24 Grunstein RR, Wilcox I, Yang TS et al, Snoring and sleep apnoea in men: association with central obesity and hypertension, *Int J Obes* (1993) **17**:533–40.

25 Leech J, Onal E, Bauer P, Lopata M, Determinants of hypercapnia in occlusive sleep apnea syndrome, *Chest* (1987) **92**:807–13.

26 Nowbar S, Burkart KM, Zwillich CW, Hypoventilation among obese patients: a common and under-diagnosed problem, *Am J Resp Crit Care Med* (2000) **161**:A890.

27 Young T, Palta M, Dempsey J et al, Occurrence of sleep disordered breathing among middle-aged adults, *N Engl J Med* (1993) **328**:1230–5.

28 Bearpark H, Elliott L, Grunstein RR et al, Snoring and sleep apnea; a population study in Australian men, *Am J Resp Crit Care Med* (1995) **151**:1459–65.

29 Pillar G, Peled R, Lavie P, Recurrence of sleep apnea without concomitant weight increase 7.5 years after weight reduction surgery, *Chest* (1994) **106**:1702–4.

30 Grunstein RR, Ho KY, Sullivan CE, Sleep apnea and acromegaly, *Ann Intern Med* (1991) **115**:527–32.

31 Sin DD, Fitzgerald F, Parker JD et al, Risk factors for central and obstructive sleep apnoea in 450 men and women with congestive heart failure, *Am J Resp Crit Care Med* (1999) **160**:1101–6.

32 Peppard PE, Young TB, Palta M, Skatrud J, Prospective study of the association between sleep-disordered breathing and hypertension, *N Engl J Med* (2000) **342**:1378–84.

33 Bearpark H, Grustein RR, Touyz S et al, Cognitive and psychological dysfunction in sleep apnoea before and after treatment with CPAP, *Sleep Res* (1987) **17**:303.

34 Brooks D, Horner RL, Kozor KF et al, Obstructive sleep apnoea as a cause of systemic hypertension. Evidence from a canine model, *J Clin Invest* (1997) **99**:106–9.

35 Fletcher EC, Bao G, Li R, Renin activity and blood pressure in response to chronic episodic hypoxia, *Hypertension* (1999) **34**:309–14.

36 Nieto FJ, Young TB, Lind BK et al, Association of sleep-disordered breathing, sleep apnea and hypertension in a large community-based study, *JAMA* (2000) **283**:1829–36.

37 Hung J, Whitford EG, Parsons RW, Hillman DR, Association of sleep apnoea and myocardial infarction in men, *Lancet* (1990) **336**:261–4.

38 Laks L, Lehrhaft B, Grunstein RR, Sullivan CE, Pulmonary hypertension in obstructive sleep apnoea, *Eur Resp J* (1995) **8**:537–41.

39 He J, Kryger M, Zorick F et al, Mortality and apnea index in obstructive sleep apnea. Experience in 385 patients, *Chest* (1988) **94**:9–14.

40 Chin K, Shimizu K, Nakamura T et al, Changes in intra-abdominal visceral fat and leptin levels in patients with OSA syndrome following nasal CPAP, *Circulation* (1999) **100**:706–12.

41 O'Donnell CP, Schaub CD, Berkowitz DE et al, Leptin prevents respiratory depression in obesity, *Am J Resp Crit Care Med* (1999) **159**:1477–84.

42 Smith PL, Gold AR, Meyers DA et al, Weight loss in mildly to moderately obese patients with obstructive sleep apnea, *Ann Intern Med* (1985) **103**:850–5.

43 Sullivan CE, Issa FG, Berthon-Jones M, Eves L, Reversal of obstructive sleep apnoea by continuous positive airway pressure applied through the nares, *Lancet* (1981) **i**:862–5.

44 Sullivan CE, Grunstein RR, Continuous positive airway pressure in sleep disordered breathing. In: Kryger MH, Dement WC, Roth TP, eds, *Principles and Practice of Sleep Disorders Medicine* (WB Saunders: Philadelphia, 1994) 559–70.

45 Jenkinson C, Davies RJ, Mullins R, Sradling JR, Comparison of therapeutic and subtherapeutic nasal continuous positive airway pressure for obstructive sleep apnoea: a randomised prospective parallel trial, *Lancet* (1999) **353**:2100–5.

46 Engleman HM, Kingshott RN, Wraith PK et al, Randomized placebo-controlled crossover trial of CPAP for mild sleep apnoea–hypopnoea syndrome, *Am J Resp Crit Care Med* (1999) **159**:461–7.

47 Millman RP, Rosenberg CL, Kramer NR, Oral appliances in the treatment of snoring and sleep apnoea, *Clin Chest Med* (1998) **19**:69–75.

48 Ryan CF, Lowe LL, Unpredictable results of laser assisted uvulopalatoplasty in the treatment of obstructive sleep apnoea, *Thorax* (2000) **55**:399–404.

49 Powell NB, Riley RW, Robinson A, Surgical management of OSA syndrome, *Clin Chest Med* (1998) **19**:77–86.

Management Approaches

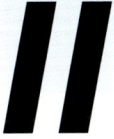

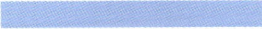

II

Dietary management of obesity

Clare M Grace

7

Helping patients make permanent, healthy changes to their eating habits is an essential component in the multidisciplinary approach to the prevention and treatment of overweight and obesity.

Although many health professionals recognize the importance of dietary management, research suggests that difficulty often arises in the translation of general nutritional messages into specific food changes, which are practical and realistic for patients to implement over the longer term.[1] Such difficulty may be related to inadequate training in nutrition and dietetics; a subject which rarely receives sufficient attention in undergraduate and postgraduate education, particularly among the medical profession.[2] Even fewer health professionals have received training which specifically addresses the knowledge and skills required for the management of the overweight and obese.

This chapter outlines the principles of dietary management in overweight and obese adults, the various treatment approaches available and, importantly, provides practical guidance on helping patients make, and sustain, healthier food choices.

Is dieting a pointless exercise?

Before considering the various processes involved in dietary management it is perhaps useful to consider the question, is dieting a worthwhile treatment strategy?

There are some who lobby against dieting, claiming that its long-term efficacy is poor and that the psychological and physical effects of weight regain outweigh the potential benefits of weight loss.[3] Indeed, it is commonly said that 90% of 'slimming' diets fail.[4] Conveying the message 'diets don't work' is not helpful to the obese and overweight population as it implies body weight is managed by forces entirely beyond the individual's control. Furthermore, it may tempt some towards 'alternative', potentially damaging methods of weight control.

Much of the condemnation of current dietary treatment strategies is based on the results of clinical trials and hospital-based programmes. Patients who participate in these represent a very small percentage of the total obese population and tend to be the more challenging patients, often presenting with significant psychological problems and a higher incidence of 'binge eating' disorder, factors known to affect treatment outcome detrimentally.[5]

It is therefore inappropriate to consider the findings from clinical trials and hospital-based programmes as being representative of the likely outcome of intervention in the general overweight and obese population.

Evaluating the long-term effect of dietary intervention is essential if we are to achieve improved practice and treatment outcomes. It has been suggested that this should be a research priority in the primary care setting.[6] Nevertheless, careful and appropriate interpretation of findings is paramount.

Interpretation of the 'diets don't work' message is also influenced by the definition of the term 'diet'; it is important to make the distinction between medically approved healthy diets with a scientific rationale and the plethora of popular weight loss diets, which often make unrealistic and scientifically unsupported claims.

Energy balance

It is well known that the body's fat and energy stores are determined by the balance between energy intake and energy expenditure. As illustrated in Figure 7.1, weight loss occurs when the body is in negative energy balance, as fat stores must be mobilized in order to meet the body's energy demands.

Negative energy balance can be induced by a reduction in energy consumed, an increase in energy expended, or a combination of both. In theory, reducing fat stores should be simple; eat less and exercise more. However, as our understanding of obesity has increased so it has become evident that the condition is not simply the result of eating too much and exercising too little. The regulation of body weight is controlled by a complex, and as yet incompletely understood, number of physiological processes which interact with various environmental and societal factors.

Dietary management

The following chapter describes the various strategies which can be used in the dietary management of obesity together with practical guidance for patients (outlined as practice points in Tables 7.2, 7.4–7.8 and 7.13). It is

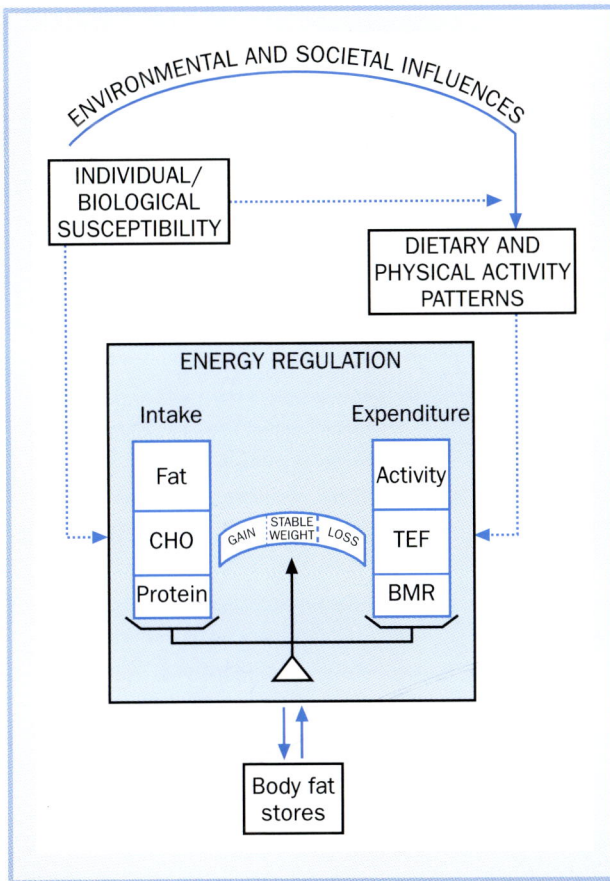

Figure 7.1
Energy balance and the physiological regulation of body weight. This figure shows the fundamental principles of energy balance and regulation. Positive energy balance occurs when energy intake is greater than energy expenditure and promotes weight gain. Conversely, negative energy balance promotes a decrease in body fat stores and weight loss. Body weight is regulated by a series of physiological processes which have the capacity to maintain weight within a relatively narrow range (stable weight). It is thought that the body exerts a stronger defence against undernutrituion and weight loss than it does against overconsumption and weight gain. TEF = thermic effect of food; BMR = basal metabolic rate; CHO = carbohydrate. Reproduced with kind permission of the World Health Organization.

not the intention of this chapter to suggest that *all* areas must be discussed with *every* patient; rather it is the clinician's responsibility to judge, through assessment and discussion with their patient, which strategies are relevant and to provide information and guidance in an appropriately staged manner. Time and financial limitations are often barriers to the management of obesity; frequent but short visits with good quality advice, the increased use of group therapy and appropriate referrals to other members of the multidisciplinary team (nurse, dietitian, psychologist) may be helpful in distributing the management workload.

How dietary management has changed over time

Traditional dietary management centres on educating patients about healthier food choices and persuading them that such changes to lifestyle are important. However, it is now recognized that simply providing nutrition education or 'prescribing' a diet is inadequate and in recent years there has been greater focus on the need to combine nutrition information with behavioural techniques.[7–9] This has resulted in an increased emphasis on *how* to implement recommended food changes.

Example If a patient regularly eats large amounts of chocolate, traditionally our advice

would be to reduce the amount of chocolate eaten and to try and convince the patient this was an important change. However, many patients are already aware that this is necessary, but their difficulty arises in implementing the advice. The modern approach would be to examine the behaviour associated with the large quantities of chocolate consumed, to look for example at the food environment and the thought processes which may trigger overconsumption, to combine this with nutrition information and to develop strategies which may help the patient to modify their behaviour, so achieving the goal of reduced chocolate consumption (refer to Chapter 8 for further details).

As weight management strategies have moved away from achieving ideal body weight towards moderate weight loss, and maintenance of this loss, so emphasis in dietary management has changed from very severe energy restrictions towards modest, staged changes which are more feasible to maintain long term. The practice of advising a fixed energy allowance, for example 1200 kcal/day, to *all* obese individuals has been subject to some criticism. The more obese the person, the higher their energy requirements and the greater the energy deficit imposed, so the more likely the person is to struggle with such drastic food changes. It has been demonstrated that compliance to dietary advice and sustained weight loss are improved with a modest deficit of 500 kcal per day (from energy requirements) compared to very severe energy restriction.[10]

Assessment

Obese and overweight patients present with very different management problems and unravelling the specific factors which are contributing to the individual's difficulty controlling weight, and which of these factors it is feasible for the patient to modify, is an important aspect of the assessment process.

The aim of assessment is to help the clinician gain an understanding of the patient's current circumstances, the possible problems they face, together with present and previous approaches to weight management

This provides insight into whether they acknowledge, and are ready to implement long-term changes to lifestyle, or whether they seek the elusive quick-fix solution to obesity (refer to Chapter 8). Information gleaned through the assessment process may help the clinician match treatments to individual patients.

Such discussions also provide an opportunity to educate patients on why some of the 'alternative' weight loss methods may not be the most effective or healthy approach to long-term weight management.

Example questions to consider:

(1) Which diets have you tried previously to lose weight?

Consider:

Have they primarily tried fad diets, quick-fix solutions or more sensible approaches. Their response to this question may help build a picture of attitudes and experiences of weight loss and whether they have made many previous attempts to control weight.

(2) How much weight did you lose with these diets and did you manage to keep this weight off long term?

Consider:

Have previous attempts centred on rapid weight loss, ie do they have unrealistic expectations of the amount of weight they can lose each week? It may be helpful to find out what they believe is an acceptable weekly weight loss.

(3) What is the longest period of time you have managed to sustain changes to your diet?

Consider:

Again this may give further insight into their approach to changing their eating habits and whether they seek the quick-fix solution. It may also provide an opportunity to discuss some of the possible barriers encountered in previous attempts at changing eating habits.

(4) Of the different diets that you may have tried previously which did you find the easiest to comply with?

Consider:

Possible indicators of the type of approach which has most suited their lifestyle. For example, have they responded best to group programmes or do they prefer an individual approach? Have they found approaches which provide more guidance on portion sizes useful or do they find systems which involve counting points or units difficult to integrate into their lifestyle?

(5) Can you think of any reasons why previous attempts at changing eating habits may not have been successful?

Consider:

Potential barriers to change, eg lack of planning, time constraints, irregular work hours, price and availability of food, others sabotaging weight loss attempts. It is also worth considering whether patients exhibit 'optimism bias' – a belief that their diet is already in line with guidelines when in reality it is not so.

(6) How much influence do you believe your eating habits have on weight change?

Consider:

If the patient does not acknowledge the important role which lifestyle plays in weight management they are unlikely to be receptive to making changes to their eating and activity. Do they believe changing eating habits

is within their control? Do they take on the responsibility for making changes to their lifestyle or do they expect the clinician to provide the solution?

During the assessment process it is important to screen patients for any evidence of eating disorders. If a diagnosis is made, patients should be referred to an eating disorders unit or a clinical psychologist.

Helping patients to develop food monitoring skills

Many patients are unaware of how much, what or where they eat. Much of the food we eat can be considered forgotten food, this is particularly so with snacks, food eaten whilst watching TV or food tasted during cooking. Helping patients increase their awareness of current eating habits is an essential first step in the management process.[11] Only when they begin to recognize the eating practices which are contributing to their excess energy intake can they move towards considering where and how to make appropriate changes. Food diaries are a very useful self-monitoring tool, encourage patients to be actively involved in treatment and may give an indication of motivation.[11]

Patients should be encouraged to record everything they eat and drink for at least one week (Figure 7.2; Table 7.1) and it may be helpful to do this prior to the first

Time	With whom and/or where?	What else are you doing?	Thoughts and feelings before eating	What have you eaten and drunk?	Amount	Thoughts and feelings after eating

Figure 7.2
Eating awareness record.

Table 7.1
Guidance on completing a food diary.

- It is best to write down all food and drink as soon as you have eaten – don't wait until the end of the day as you may forget some foods and drinks. Carry the food diary with you wherever possible.
- Describe the food in detail, eg rather than just writing a chicken sandwich, record:
    how many slices of bread, the type of bread
    the type of spread used, whether it was spread thickly or thinly
    the number of slices of chicken in the sandwich
    whether mayonnaise/salad dressing was used, which type (brand name)
- Write the amounts of foods/drink you have, either in weights ie grammes (g) or ounces (oz) or simple household measures, eg:
    1 glass = 200 ml
    1 cup = 150 ml
    4 tablespoons of branflakes
    1 large slice of wholemeal bread
- Record the method of cooking, eg fried, grilled, boiled or baked.
- It can also be helpful to consider the circumstances associated with eating. Consider the time you ate, where you were when you ate and how you felt before and after eating. Can you identify any factors which trigger eating?

appointment. Some patients choose to keep continuous food diaries as a method of aiding compliance to newly adopted eating habits. Interestingly, research into those who have lost and successfully maintained their lowered weight for at least 2 years has found regular self-monitoring to be a common feature.[12]

Restarting a food diary if weight loss is not proceeding as planned may also prove a useful strategy. The process of completing a food diary is often sufficient for many patients to begin acknowledging where changes are required. Consider and discuss the various issues outlined below with patients to help build a picture of the behaviours and factors contributing to their difficulties in managing weight.

Issues to consider include:

- *Timing of meals* Were meals skipped? If so why was this? Was this a conscious weight loss technique by the patient or was this related to time or organization issues? Were they grazing throughout the day? Were they eating snacks rather than meals? Were they eating late at night or during the night?
- *Speed of eating* How fast was the patient eating? Did they notice they had finished their meal before anyone else? Did they taste and enjoy the food they were eating? Were they bingeing? (refer to Chapter 8.)
- *Place of eating* Where were they when they were eating? Were they at home or eating out? Were they seated at a table, in front of the TV or elsewhere? Do they eat significantly more or less while with others? Do their patterns of eating change significantly at weekends?

- *Other activities* Were they doing anything else while eating? Were they watching TV, reading a book, driving the car?
- *Emotional connections* How did they feel before and after eating? Could they link any particular feelings or emotions to overeating. Did they experience food cravings?

The food diary can be used as the basis for discussion so specific food changes can be agreed between clinician and patient. However, it is important that such discussions are conducted in a sensitive and nonjudgmental way.

Under-reporting of energy intake

Although food diaries are a very useful self-monitoring tool it is important to recognize that they are very unlikely to provide an accurate reflection of the patient's true energy intake. It is well recognized that under-reporting of energy intake is a common phenomenon, particularly among the overweight and obese, or those who have previously been overweight and are now 'diet conscious'.[13,14]

The reasons why people under-report

intake are poorly understood, but may be related to one or more of the following: a tendency to report a 'healthy' diet rather than actual intake or to report dieting rather than habitual behaviour, inaccurate recording due to memory lapses or the time-consuming or inconvenient nature of the task results in poor record keeping.[15]

Patients who seem unable to lose weight while reporting energy intakes of 1000 kcal or less per day are almost certainly under-reporting their true intake. In such circumstances it may be useful to calculate the patient's estimated energy expenditure (less a fixed deficit) and discuss dietary needs and changes based on this value (see later).

Although it is important to be aware of under-reporting, great care must be taken to ensure this information is shared with the patient in a nonjudgmental way.

Regular eating

Some patients, particularly those who have attempted to diet many times previously, often have disordered eating patterns with erratic eating times and missed meals.

Patients may skip meals as a means of controlling weight, turning to 'grazing' patterns of eating. To many it may seem logical that one less meal a day would result in quicker weight loss. However, evidence suggests the reverse; meal skipping leads to increased eating and overcompensation later

in the day and commonly to increased snacking on high fat, energy dense foods.[16] Patients who present with an irregular pattern of eating must initially focus on establishing regular meals and planned snacks (eating every 3 to 4 hours) before any attempt to lose weight.[17] It may be helpful to educate patients about why the body needs regular food and the physical and psychological effects if the body is denied fuel.

Key points in dietary management

- It is useful to emphasize the overall health benefits of eating well rather than focusing solely on weight loss effects, for example reduced risk of developing cardiovascular disease and certain cancers.

- Changing eating habits is challenging; the way people eat and what they eat are long-standing habits which cannot be changed overnight. It follows that as obesity is a chronic relapsing condition, regular support is central to successful management.[18,19]

- As health professionals we tend to talk to patients in terms of nutrients: 'it's important to reduce your fat intake'. However, patients do not make nutrient changes they make food changes, therefore it is vital that such nutritional messages are translated into food changes pertinent to the individual which are sustainable and enjoyable.[20]

- It is often very tempting to *tell* patients what areas they should be changing in their diet. However, it is helpful to involve patients in food change decisions and, if possible, guide them towards suggesting these changes themselves.
- Be specific in food change goals. For example, rather than the goal being to eat less fatty food, which is very general, it would be preferable for the patients to set specific goals such as to eat less fatty foods by changing from butter to a low-fat spread and to use fat-free salad dressings rather than mayonnaise in salads and sandwiches. This focuses the patient on exactly which behaviours they are going to change, rather than the previously rather vague target.
- Do not expect or suggest all changes to be made at the same time. A staged approach is often the most appropriate, starting with two or three key changes. Once these have been adopted and accepted, further changes can be agreed.
- In ensuring that dietary changes are practical for the patient to implement, consider and discuss time constraints, financial limitations, cooking ability and facilities as well as making sure the diet remains palatable and enjoyable.
- Involving partners and families in the patient's attempts to make healthier choices is important in increasing compliance to dietary changes and as a

cost effective means of extending health messages.[21] It seems that including partners in the management programme helps through continued reinforcement of treatment strategies and increased attendance rates.[22,23] Gaining support and developing helping relationships with family and friends is important to the patient's goal of staying committed to being a healthy eater.

- For some patients the word 'diet' conveys messages of deprivation, avoidance of favourite foods and the need to eat small portions of foods they do not enjoy.[24] Furthermore, it is often considered to be something which only needs to be followed until the desired weight loss has been achieved, after which it can be abandoned and the very eating habits which contributed to excess weight resumed. Patients need to understand that as obesity is a chronic condition so weight control will require life-long attention, and as such the lifestyle strategies they use to achieve their lowered weight have to be acceptable for the longer term.

Different treatment strategies

There are a variety of approaches which can be used to help patients adopt a healthier way of eating. These can be crudely divided into qualitative approaches which focus on changing the type of foods eaten using general healthy eating guidelines, versus more structured quantitative approaches which give specific details of quantities and portion sizes of foods.

It is now recognized that no one (dietary) approach or method of delivery will suit all patients, rather each method may be appropriate for some patients but not others.[25] This will depend on the patient's previous dieting experience, current eating habits and lifestyle. For example, some patients may have been given healthy eating advice previously and found it useful but not specific enough and they may wish for greater direction with regard to portion sizes. For others, such specific guidance or the need to count or measure food is unnecessary or unhelpful and focusing on healthy eating principles, substituting high-fat for low-fat foods, may be a more suitable approach.

Gone are the days of giving the same 'standard' diet sheet to all patients with the expectation of this leading to weight loss. Meal plans, which lay out precisely what should be eaten each day, allow no flexibility for eating out or social events and do nothing to re-educate eating habits.

General guidance on healthy eating

The principles of healthy eating relevant to weight loss are:
- Eat plenty of foods rich in starch and fibre
- Eat plenty of fruit and vegetables
- Avoid eating too much fat
- Do not eat sugary foods too often
- Keep alcohol within sensible limits

Scientific rationale behind these guidelines

It is helpful to understand the scientific basis of recommended nutrient changes and the evidence relating to the proposed influence of the various macronutrients (protein, carbohydrate and fat) on energy balance.

Why less fat?

There is good evidence to support the association between dietary fat intake and increasing obesity. Certainly, over the last 50 years as the prevalence of obesity has increased, the carbohydrate content of our diet has fallen while the fat content has risen dramatically.[26,27]

Fat appears to exert its greatest influence on energy balance through its effects on appetite. In studies where people have been allowed to eat as much as they like, the same quantity of food is generally eaten with high fat as with high carbohydrate meals, but because fat gram for gram contains more than twice the number of calories as carbohydrate, considerably more calories are consumed.[28] This phenomenon is often termed 'passive overconsumption'. Various metabolic studies have shown that the body is more efficient at digesting and storing fat compared to other macronutrients, with very little wastage of energy during processing. It is also the nutrient which fails to produce a compensatory increase in oxidation if intake is increased. In contrast, the body appears to be well programmed to oxidize protein and carbohydrate in preference to fat, so an increase in carbohydrate intake will lead to a measurable increase in carbohydrate oxidation.

Why more carbohydrate?

Carbohydrate is known to have a greater satiating effect than fat and its intake is quite closely regulated by the body.[29] Furthermore, high carbohydrate meals appear to keep hunger suppressed for longer than meals high in fat.[30]

Whether the type of carbohydrate influences energy balance has been subject to some debate. The energy density (calories per unit weight) of carbohydrate varies depending on the type of carbohydrate, for example bread has a lower energy density than sugar. Evidence is beginning to emerge which supports the theory that low energy density carbohydrates tend to result in lower energy intakes than high energy density carbohydrates,[31] so supporting the increased consumption of high fibre starchy carbohydrates rather than simple sugars to replace fats.

Why more fruits and vegetables?

Fruits and vegetables are naturally low in fat, high in fibre and are rich sources of vitamins and minerals, particularly antioxidant nutrients such as vitamin C, beta-carotene, selenium and others such as lycopene.

Epidemiological studies suggest the antioxidant and fibre content of fruit and vegetables provides protection against disease, particularly cardiovascular disease and cancer.[32] The mechanism behind this protective effect is believed to be the capacity of antioxidants to scavenge free radicals, preventing DNA damage and subsequent mutation and decreasing atherosclerosis.[33,34]

Why moderate alcohol?

Alcohol seems to bypass the body's appetite regulation system with no apparent compensation for its energy content by reduction in energy from food.[35] Furthermore, alcohol will be oxidized in preference to other nutrients, so increasing the tendency towards fat storage.[36]

Getting the message across

The National Food Guide, 'The balance of good health',[37–39] is a pictorial method which was developed to help convey healthy eating messages and is based on the government's guidelines for a healthy diet (Figure 7.3). It

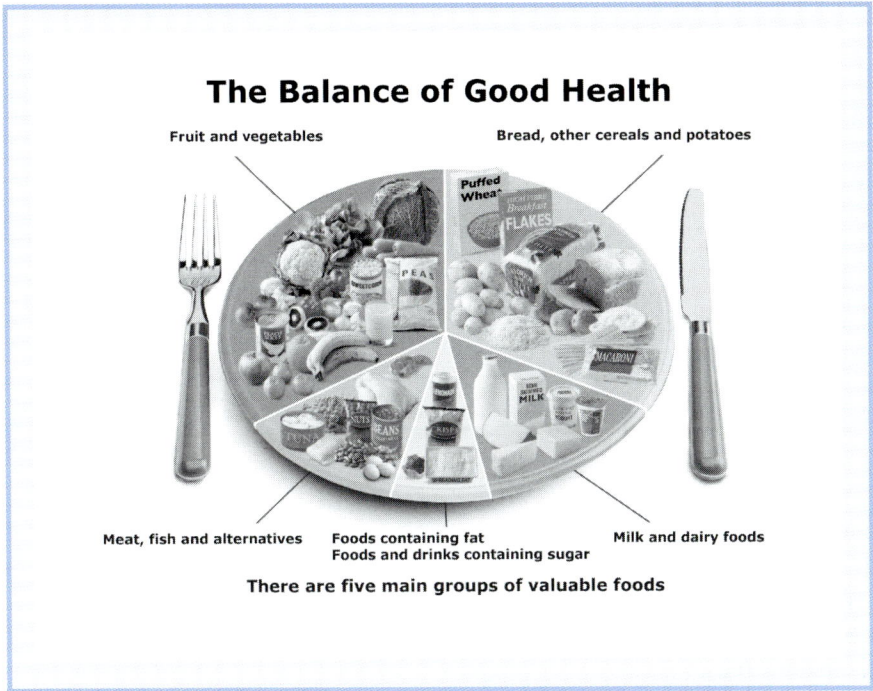

Figure 7.3
The Balance of Good Health. Printed with kind permission of the Food Standards Agency.

uses pictures of food and drink rather than nutritional 'jargon' to demonstrate balanced food choices, and may be easier for patients to understand than unfamiliar terms such as calories or nutrient groups.

The model divides food into five food groups and the size of the plate divisions represents the balance of foods needed to make up a healthy diet. It emphasizes the large contribution of fruit and vegetables, the need to increase starchy foods and the importance of limiting, although not removing completely, foods high in sugars and fat.

This method can be used as an attractive teaching tool, or form the basis of discussion, and may aid recall on the required food changes and a balanced diet.

The five food groups

(1) Bread, other cereals and potatoes
(2) Fruit and vegetables
(3) Meat, fish and alternatives
(4) Milk and dairy foods
(5) Fatty and sugary foods

Using each food group as the basis for discussion, healthy food choices specific to that patient can be agreed. Tables 7.2, 7.4–7.8 and 7.13 summarize possible changes to consider with each patient.

Bread, other cereals, potatoes (Table 7.2)

These foods are major sources of starchy carbohydrate, nonstarch polysaccharide (fibre), B vitamins, calcium and iron. Many people believe starchy foods are fattening and often avoid, or limit, their consumption. Increasing starchy foods is the mainstay of healthy eating for the reasons previously outlined. To help patients dispel the myth of starch being fattening it is important to explain that the extra fat added to these foods is the source of excess calories, rather than starch per se, for example the creamy rich sauce with pasta, the knob of butter on a jacket potato or the oil used to fry potatoes.

Fruit and vegetables (Tables 7.3 and 7.4)

These are very good sources of vitamins, particularly antioxidant vitamins, minerals and nonstarch polysaccharide (fibre), are naturally low in fat and should form an important part of any healthy diet. Unfortunately, most people fall short on their

Table 7.2
How to eat more starchy foods.

Practice points
• Increase the amount of starchy foods (bread, rice, pasta, potatoes) on your plate
• Try a high-fibre breakfast cereal such as Weetabix, Fruit and Fibre, branflakes, Shredded wheat or porridge
• Bread, pasta, rice and potatoes are not fattening. It is the fat that often goes with these foods that may contribute to weight gain, eg the cheese sauce with pasta, the liberal spreading of butter on bread and the oil used to fry potatoes. Try wholemeal bread, brown rice and whole-wheat pasta
• Tea cakes, currant buns and plain biscuits are a healthier choice than rich cakes and biscuits, but avoid adding extra butter, margarine or spread to these foods and remember they are not calorie free.

Table 7.3
What is a fruit/vegetable portion?

> *1 portion is*
>   *2 tbsp vegetables*
>   *1 small bowl of salad*
>   *1 piece of fruit*
>   *2 tbsp stewed or tinned fruit*
>   *100 ml fruit juice*

Meat, fish and alternatives (Table 7.5)

The food items in this group include meat, poultry, fish, beans, eggs and nuts. These foods are valuable sources of protein, iron, B vitamins, zinc and magnesium, however care must be taken to ensure they are not high in fat. Red meat has received a great deal of bad press over recent years, resulting in many people believing it to be an unhealthy food which should be avoided. However, red meat can be part of a healthy diet so long as lean cuts are chosen and it is cooked in a low-fat way. When discussing this food group with patients, emphasize the importance of making low-fat choices.

intake. It is a good idea to discuss with patients the importance of eating the recommended five portions of fruit and vegetables each day and how best to achieve this.

Table 7.4
How to eat more fruit.

> *Practice points*
> - *Try to follow the 'five a day' guide*
> - *Slice a banana or apple on your breakfast cereal or add grapes or strawberries*
> - *Have a side salad with your main meal*
> - *Keep a fruit bowl on your desk at work*
> - *Buy an exotic fruit, eg mango, kiwi, rather than a chocolate bar*
> - *Chop fruit into yoghurt or sugar-free jelly*
> - *Keep plenty of frozen vegetables in the freezer and add extra to soups, stews and casseroles*
> - *Choose unsweetened fruit juice and have a small glass a day in place of a piece of fruit*
> - *Use tinned fruit in natural juice rather than in syrup*
> - *Have a fruit salad as a dessert either at home or in a restaurant*

Table 7.5
How to eat lean protein foods.

Practice points
- *Watch out for fat!*
- *Choose lean cuts of meat*
- *Trim all visible fat from meat before cooking and remove skin from chicken and turkey*
- *Cook joints of meat and poultry on an oven rack so fat can drip through. Do not use this fat to baste, instead try using stock or cover with foil to retain juices*
- *After cooking stews and casseroles allow them to cool and skim off any excess fat*
- *Try to eat chicken, turkey, fish and beans more frequently than red meat. There is no need to 'cut out' red meat, it can be part of a healthy diet but it is important to choose lean cuts*
- *Use beans and pulses such as baked beans, chick peas, lentils and kidney beans. Add to soups, stews and salads*
- *As you increase the starchy foods on your plate reduce the amount of meat, fish or chicken*
- *Remember nuts are high in fat and calories so try to eat them in moderation*
- *Shellfish and fish are low in fat but be careful about how they've been cooked. If they are in batter, marinated in oil, or covered in a rich sauce they will be high in fat*
- *Watch out for added fat in egg dishes, eg egg mayonnaise or fried eggs*

Milk and dairy foods (Table 7.6)

Food items included in this group include milk, cheese and yoghurt. These foods are important sources of protein, vitamins A, D, E and B_{12} and minerals, particularly calcium, but unless low-fat options are chosen they can contribute significant amounts of fat to the diet. In an attempt to reduce their calorie intake, some overweight and obese patients may, rather than use low-fat alternatives, avoid dairy foods completely. This may result in a diet low in essential vitamins and minerals and such patients should be guided to reintroduce low-fat dairy foods to their diet.

Fats and sugars (Table 7.7)

This group includes:

- Foods containing fat: margarine, butter, other spreading fats, low-fat spreads, oils, oily salad dressings, salad cream, mayonnaise, cream, chocolate, crisps, biscuits, pastries, cake, puddings, ice cream, rich sauces and gravies.
- Foods containing sugar: soft drinks, sweets, jam, cake, puddings, biscuits, pastries and ice cream.

There are three different kinds of fats: saturated, monounsaturated and

Table 7.6
How to eat lower-fat dairy foods.

> **Practice points**
> - *Choose skimmed or semi-skimmed milk rather than whole milk*
> - *Swap full-fat yoghurt for low-fat natural yoghurt or diet fruit-flavoured yoghurt or fromage frais*
> - *Be careful with cheese. Even small amounts of cheese contain large amounts of fat. Limit intake of hard cheese, even half fat hard cheese*
> - *Try to avoid nibbling on chunks of cheese in-between meals*
> - *Use low-fat cheese spreads and cottage cheese in preference to hard cheese*
> - *Try yoghurt as a replacement for ice cream or desserts*

Table 7.7
How to eat less fat.

> **Practice points**
> - *Spread less fat on your bread. Ideally choose low-fat spreads rather than margarine or butter and use sparingly*
> - *Choose cooking methods that do not need the addition of oil or fat. Try boiling, steaming, microwaving and grilling. If oil is used, limit the quantity by measuring with a teaspoon and then reducing the number of teaspoons used, or try an oil spray*
> - *Avoid the unnecessary addition of fat and/or oil to food, ie butter, margarine or low-fat spread to potatoes or vegetables, butter used on bread for beans on toast or soup, or sandwiches with moist fillings*
> - *Limit pastries, cakes, chocolates and crisps but do not think of them as bad foods which cannot be eaten*
> - *Swap mayonnaise, salad cream and French/vinaigrette type dressings for fat-free or oil-free alternatives or use low-fat yoghurt-based dressings or lemon juice and vinegar*
> - *Try an artificial sweetener in drinks and cooking*
> - *Swap sugary fizzy drinks for diet versions and try a sugar-free diluting squash in place of the full-sugar version*
> - *Sauces usually contain butter or margarine, but it is possible to make them from milk, cornflour and seasoning. If you use jars or packets of 'cook-in' sauces avoid those which contain cream or cheese. Tomato-based sauces are a better choice*

polyunsaturated. It is well known that diets which contain large amounts of saturated fat are associated with an increased risk of heart disease, hence the recommendation to reduce the amount of saturated fat eaten and to use monounsaturated fats instead.

However, it is important to emphasize that the overall aim, when managing weight, is the reduction of the *total* fats. This message is commonly misinterpreted by patients; olive oil is rich in monounsaturates and is certainly preferable to using lard; however, although it is a 'healthier' fat, using large amounts of olive oil will have the same effect on weight as lard. It would be better to change the way foods are cooked so the addition of fat can be avoided, but whenever fat is essential small amounts of oil can be used.

Chief sources of saturated fat include: fatty meats, meat products such as sausages and burgers, hard cheese, butter, hydrogenated margarine, pastry and cakes. Chief sources of monounsaturates include: rapeseed, olive oil and olive oil spreads.

Many obese and overweight patients perceive high-fat snack foods (for example crisps, chocolate, cakes, biscuits) to be 'forbidden foods' that should be 'cut out' completely if weight loss is to occur. Banning foods and striving for the 'perfect diet' can be counterproductive. It tends to lead to

increased cravings for such foods and, following their consumption, feelings of guilt, which in turn can lead to further 'comfort eating'. Crisps, chocolates, cakes and biscuits can be part of a healthy diet so long as the amounts and frequency of consumption are limited.

Alcohol (Table 7.8)

For general health purposes it is recommended that alcohol is kept within sensible limits. Women are advised to keep to 2 to 3 units or less per day, and men between 3 and 4 units or less per day.

A unit of alcohol =
$\frac{1}{2}$ pint beer or lager (300 ml)
1 glass of wine (125 ml)
1 pub measure of spirit
1 medium glass of sherry (50 ml)

However for those trying to lose weight it may be necessary to limit alcohol further for the reasons outlined previously.

Table 7.8
How to reduce alcohol.

Practice points
- *Try alternating alcoholic drinks with soft, low-calorie drinks*
- *Be careful about drinking fruit juice or standard soft drinks instead of alcohol as they tend to be high in calories*
- *Drink half pints rather than pints. Dilute spirits or wine with low-calorie soft drinks or fizzy water and make the drink last for more than one round*
- *Don't drink low-alcohol beers and wines in the belief they are lower in calories as they tend to contain large amounts of sugar*

The Balance of Good Health brain teaser

Try assessing your patient's understanding of how to apply 'The Balance of Good Health' practically using the test illustrated in Figure 7.4 and described in Tables 7.9 and 7.10.

Although changing the type and balance of foods eaten may be sufficient for many to lose weight, some patients may wish for further guidance on quantities and portion sizes. 'The Balance of Good Health' does not usually specify portion sizes as every individual has different needs and unless health professionals are confident in determining patient requirements and translating these into specific portion sizes, ranges of portion sizes can be misleading and inappropriate.

Guidelines on individual energy needs and portion sizes

Further guidelines on how to calculate individual energy needs and translate these

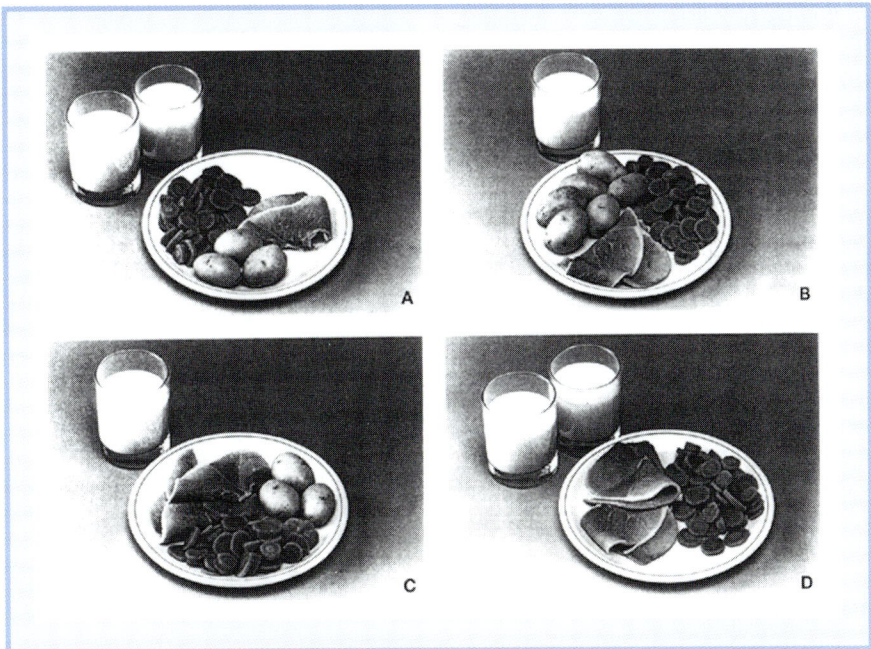

Figure 7.4
The Balance of Good Health brain teaser. Printed with kind permission of the Food Standards Agency.

Table 7.9
'The Balance of Good Health' brain teaser.

Figure 7.4 is a meal made up of the same foods but in different proportions. One of the meals is more healthy than the other four and one less healthy.

(1) Which of the four photographs is the more healthy of the four? Why?
(2) Which of the four photographs is the less healthy of the four? Why?
(3) What changes could be made to any of the other three to make them more healthy?

Answers in Table 7.10.

Table 7.10
Answers for 'The Balance of Good Health' brain teaser.

Answers
All meals contain a large portion of carrots, but vegetables can only be considered truly 'healthy' if eaten in the correct proportion and balance with other foods

(1) B is the healthiest as it contains twice as much 'veg' and 'potato' to 'meat' and 'milk'.
(2) D is the least healthy as it contains no bread, cereal or potato
(3) Add or increase the amount of potato or other starchy foods in A, C and D. Reduce the portion of meat in C and D.

Nutritional composition
B – 1 slice of ham, 6 potatoes, large carrots, standard glass of milk = 357 kcal, 17% energy from fat
A – 1 slice of ham, 3 potatoes, large carrots, large milk = 359 kcal, 24% energy from fat
C – 2 slices ham, 3 potatoes, large carrots, standard glass of milk = 324 kcal, 25% energy from fat
D – 2 slices ham, no potatoes, large carrots, large milk = 326 kcal, 32% fat

---

into specific portion sizes for each patient are outlined below.

Quantitative approaches

One quantitative approach which may be used is an individually designed weight loss plan as outlined by the Scottish Intercollegiate Guidelines Network.[40] This involves the calculation of a patient's energy allowance which is then translated into units or exchanges which are chosen from six food groups. Such detail on portion sizes can be beneficial for some obese patients.

Calculating energy prescription (Table 7.11)

Using the equation appropriate for the patient's age, gender, height (m) and weight (kg), calculate the basal metabolic rate. Multiply the BMR value by a physical activity factor of 1.3 (sedentary lifestyle), which will give the patient's total energy requirements. To allow the patient to lose 1–2 lb per week (equivalent to ~3500 kcal) subtract 500–600 kcal from total energy requirements to produce the final daily calorie allowance.

Example

A female patient, age 33, weight 90 kg, height 1.65 m

$$BMR = 8.7 \times 90 - 25 \times 1.65 + 865$$
$$= 1607 \text{ kcal} \times 1.3$$
$$= 2089 \text{ kcal}$$

subtract 600

Gives a daily calorie allowance of 1500 kcal per day

Table 7.11
How to predict basal metabolic rate (BMR).

	Age range (years)	BMR (kcal) (kJ in parentheses)
Men	18–30	15.4 W − 27 H + 717 (64.4 W − 113 H + 3000)
	30–60	11.3 W + 16 H + 901 (47.2 W + 66.9 H + 3769)
	>60	8.8 W + 1128 H − 1071 (36.8 W + 4719.5 H − 4481)
Women	18–30	13.3 W + 334 H + 35 (55.6 W + 1397.4 H + 146)
	30–60	8.7 W − 25 H + 865 (36.4 W − 104.6 H + 3619)
	>60	9.2 W + 637 H − 302 (38.5 W + 2665.2 H − 1264)

W = weight; H = height.

Now look at Table 7.12 which translates the calorie prescription into exchanges allocated for each food group. The quantities which constitute an exchange for each food group are outlined in Table 7.13. It will be necessary to take some time to explain to patients how the system can be used in practice.

A 1500 kcal diet translates into:

6 starch points

2 fruit points

5 meat points

4 fat points

2 milk points

and ~150 extra calories per day

After modest weight losses of ≥5 kg a further reduction of ~300 kcal in the energy prescription may be required if weight has slowed or plateaued and further weight loss is desired.[40] Energy prescriptions should not be taken below 1200 kcal/day.

What if no weight loss occurs with lifestyle intervention?

For some patients low-fat, healthy eating advice, no matter how individually tailored, does not result in weight loss. If an adequate trial period, 3 to 6 months, of lifestyle

Table 7.12
Energy–food exchange.

Energy prescription	Starch	Fruit	Meat	Fat	Milk	Veg	Allowance for extras (kcal)
1200	5	2	4	3	1.5	3	115
1300	5	2	4	4	1.5	4	145
1400	5	2	5	4	2	4	145
1500	6	2	5	4	2	4	165
1600	6	3	6	4	2	4	150
1700	7	3	6	5	2	4	125
1800	7	3	7	5	2	5	145
1900	8	3	7	5	2	5	165
2000	8	4	8	5	2	5	150
2100	9	4	8	6	2	5	125
2200	9	4	9	6	2.5	5	125
2300	10	4	9	6	2.5	5	145
2400	10	5	9	7	2.5	5	140
2500	11	5	9	7	2.5	5	160
2600	12	5	9	8	2.5	5	135
2700	12	5	10	8	2.5	6	155
2800	13	5	10	8	3	6	130

Table 7.13
How to make healthier choices when eating out.

- *If possible discuss with the waiter or chef how various foods on the menu have been prepared and let them know you are following a low-fat healthy diet. Ask for your food without oil, butter/margarine, rich sauces or pastry*
- *Try light starters, eg melon, grapefruit, Parma ham, soup*
- *It is usually possible to swap chips or fries for jacket or boiled potatoes and to have vegetables without butter or sauce*
- *For main course try grilled meat or fish with salad or plenty of vegetables*
- *Request salad dressings, gravies and sauces to be served on the side and use only a small amount*
- *Ask for low-fat milk in coffee rather than cream*

The following terms on menus generally suggest a suitable low-fat dish:
Au vin, baked, consommé, marinated, poached, tomato-based sauces, yoghurt sauces, stir-fried
These terms generally suggest high-fat foods:
Au gratin, basted, breaded, buttery, cheesy, creamy, crispy, en croute, hollandaise, rich, sautéed, smothered, stuffed

intervention has been allowed and limited progress has been made, a review of the entire treatment programme will be necessary. Some patients may require more specialist dietary treatment and it is suggested that such patients are referred to a state registered dietitian (SRD) nutritionist.

Other issues

Very-low-calorie diets

Very-low-calorie diets (VLCD) are formulae which provide 800 kcal or less per day together with sufficient protein, vitamins and minerals to sustain health over the short term. Although VLCDs are effective at inducing short-term weight loss the difficulty arises in the maintenance of this weight loss once patients return to conventional foods.[41] Furthermore there is some debate over the effect of VLCDs on the composition of weight lost, with the possibility of greater loss of lean tissue compared to less radical interventions.[42]

VLCDs should not be used indiscriminately and are best reserved for use in specialist obesity clinics.[43] Wherever VLCDs are used, it is essential that recommendations outlined in the Committee on Medical Aspects of Food Policy report are followed.[44] VLCDs are considered appropriate in those severely obese subjects who need to lose weight quickly for medical reasons. However, it is important to help patients recognize the need for long-term commitment to healthy food and activity changes and to follow an appropriate management programme post-VLCD.

Eating out

This is often an area of concern to patients and in those who eat out regularly it is an important area to consider. The practical suggestions in Table 7.14 and Appendix 1 may be helpful in restaurants/cafés and with 'take-away' foods.

Vegetarian diets

In recent years there has been a great increase in the number of people adopting vegetarian diets. It is often assumed products labelled vegetarian are automatically low fat and low calorie. This is not always the case, and indeed some vegetarian dishes rely heavily on the use of high-fat items such as cheese, pastry and oil. For a low-fat vegetarian diet meat items should be exchanged for dishes based on soya, quorn, tofu, beans and pulses and those including cheese, oil and pastry should be limited.

Commercially-promoted diets

The slimming industry is booming and there are many popular weight loss diets on the market. Some of these best-selling diets raise concerns: they often promote a 'quick fix' solution to obesity, may be nutritionally unsound and generally have no scientific basis to their claims. Those to be particularly wary of include: diets which advocate one food only (for example 'the grapefruit diet'), diets which ban foods (for example, 'no chocolate diet') or promote certain foods (for example 'the drinking man's diet'), food-combining approaches (for example the Hay diet), starvation diets, detox diets or low-carbohydrate diets (for example the Atkins diet).

Food labelling

There is much confusion about the true meaning of food labels and the various claims which are used to entice the consumer to choose a particular product. Unfortunately, without adequate knowledge and understanding products can be purchased in the belief they are the healthier option when in fact this may be far from the truth. It is important that health professionals are in a position to help patients understand and interpret food labels so they can compare similar products and make more informed choices.

Table 7.14
How to make healthier 'take-away' choices.

	Healthier options	Be careful with
Sandwiches	Bread, pitta, large roll Beef and pickle/mustard Ham, chicken with salad Turkey and cranberry Cottage cheese and salad Smoked salmon Low-fat cheese spread Tuna and sweetcorn	Croissant Mayonnaise Salad dressings Thickly spread butter or margarine
Café	Baked beans on toast Grilled bacon sandwich Tinned tomatoes on toast Bread muffins	Fried bacon, fried egg Cream cakes
Chinese	Chop suey dishes Beef in oyster sauce Stir-fried dishes Boiled rice	Battered dishes Duck Fried rice Prawn crackers
Indian	Tikka dish Tandoori dish Boiled rice Chappati	Korma Biriani Naan and pilau rice Samosa and bhaji
Pizza	Thick base with extra vegetables	Extra cheese Garlic bread Pepperoni Salad dressings
Burger bars	Plain burgers Salad Chicken or fish burgers	Cheese Chips Mayonnaise Milk shakes

---

The technical meaning of nutritional claims

Low fat	less than 5% fat (ie less than 5 g fat per 100 g/100 ml)
Fat free	less than 0.15% fat
Sugar free	less than 0.2% sugar
Reduced fat	a minimum of a 25% reduction in fat content

Examples of nutrition claims

85% fat free	Lite/light
Low in cholesterol	Reduced fat
No added sugar	Low fat

The nutritional claims in manufacturers' food labels are commonly misinterpreted by consumers for several reasons:

They rely on the public's limited knowledge of nutrition. A good example of this is low cholesterol claims, which exploit the public's inability to make the distinction between blood cholesterol and dietary cholesterol. Many people are unaware that the restriction of dietary cholesterol has no significant role to play in the management of hyperlipidaemia.[44] Some foods labelled 'low in cholesterol' may be high in fat and therefore not the healthiest choice for those managing their weight.

• Manufacturers can be selective in their nutrition claims. For example, a product may be labelled 'high in fibre', but although this implies a healthy item it says nothing about the overall nutritional composition and the food may also be high in fat or sugar.

• Claims that a product is 'x% fat free' are one of the most misleading labelling strategies used by manufacturers: consumers often fail to understand that 85% fat free means the product still contains 15% fat and this is no guarantee the product will be the healthiest available on the market. Furthermore, products labelled x% fat free and low fat may contain more sugar than the original item, resulting in a minimal difference in their calorie content. For example, an 85% fat free chocolate caramel bar contains 106 calories, 3.4 g fat and 20 g carbohydrate, while a comparable original chocolate caramel bar contains 125 calories, 6.4 g fat and 17 g carbohydrate – a saving of only 19 calories per bar!

• Similarly, 'reduced-fat' products, although lower in fat than the original, remain high-fat foods which still contain a considerable percentage of their calories as fat.

• 'Lite' and 'light' claims may not always be referring to the nutritional content of the product but rather to the texture or weight of the item. Even when it is a reference to the fat and calorie content, the difference may be small. For example, Lite crisps

(33% less fat) contain 135 kcal and 6.4 g fat per packet, while original crisps contain 183 kcal and 11.4 g fat per packet – a saving of 48 kcal and 5 g fat per packet.

In the light of such misleading claims, the Ministry of Agriculture, Food and Fisheries (United Kingdom) has recently revised its food labelling guidelines and suggested that x% fat free and low cholesterol claims should no longer be used by manufacturers.[45]

How can consumers compare products

In choosing the healthiest product there are two main ways of making effective comparisons:

(1) Examine the ingredients list. Ingredients are listed in descending order of quantity, so items at the beginning of the list are present in the greatest quantity. It is important to remember that fat is referred to by many different names, including triglyceride, hydrogenated vegetable fat, oil, lard, ghee, creamed coconut.

(2) Examine the nutritional information. Wherever a nutritional claim is made, manufacturers are obliged to provide relevant information. When comparing similar products, the per 100 g/100 ml section should be assessed together with some consideration of the usual portion

or serving size. Lower fat products are defined as those with a total fat content of less than 5 g per 100 g.

Group versus individual management

Group therapy offers the advantages of structure, support and competition that are not generally evident in individual therapy. It may also be more cost effective in the use of professional manpower and is an attractive option to busy general practices where there may be a large number of patients requiring weight management. Group sessions are likely to suit the more sociable patients, but for the shyer patient, individual one-to-one counselling may be a preferred option.

Conclusion

Helping patients make permanent healthy changes to their eating is a complex process, and is not simply about increasing the patient's knowledge of nutrition and diet. Rather, it requires practical information to be tailored to the patient's circumstances and for consideration to be given not only to eating behaviour but also to the reasons behind this behaviour (Chapter 8). Dietary management must be considered part of a comprehensive treatment package, which also addresses activity and behavioural issues as well as adjuncts to lifestyle management where appropriate.

References

1   Murray S, Narayan V, Mitchell M, White H, Study of dietetic knowledge among members of the primary health care team, *Br J Gen Pract* (1993) **43**:229–31.

2   Summerbell CD, Teaching nutrition to medical doctors: the potential role of the State Registered Dietitian, *J Hum Nutr Dietet* (1996) **9**:349–56.

3   Wooley SC, Garner DM, Obesity treatment: the high cost of false hope, *J Am Dietet Assoc* (1991) **91**(10):1248–51.

4   Blackburn GL, Wilson GT, Kanders BS et al, Weight cycling: the experience of human dieters, *Am J Clin Nutr* (1989) **49**:1105–9.

5   Fitzgibbon ML, Stolley MR, Kirschenbaum DS, Obese people who seek treatment have different characteristics than those who do not seek treatment, *Health Psychol* (1993) **12**:342–5.

6   Little P, Margetts B, The importance of diet and physical activity in the treatment of conditions managed in general practice, *Br J Gen Pract* (1996) **46**(404):187–92.

7   Rapoport L, Integrating cognitive behavioral therapy into dietetic practice: a challenge for dietitians, *J Hum Nutr Dietet* (1998) **11**:227–37.

8   Isselmann MC, Deubner LS, Hartman M, A nutrition counseling workshop: integrating counseling psychology into nutrition practice, *Am Dietet Assoc* (1993) **93**(3):324–6.

9   Long CG, Simpson CM, Allott EA, Psychological and dietetic counseling combined in the treatment of obesity: a comparative study in a hospital outpatient clinic, *Hum Nutr Appl Nutr* (1983) **37A**:94–102.

10   Frost G, Masters K, King C et al, A new method of energy prescription to improve weight loss, *J Hum Nutr Dietet* (1991) **4**:369–73.

11   British Dietetic Association, Obesity treatment: future directions for the contributions of dietitians, *J Hum Nutr Dietet* (1997) **10**:95–101.

12   Colvin RH, Olsen SB, A descriptive analysis of men and women who have lost significant weight and are highly successful at maintaining the loss, *Addict Behav* (1983) **8**:287–95.

13   Prentice AM, Black AE, Coward WA et al, High levels of energy expenditure in obese women, *Br Med J* (1986) **292**:983–7.

14   Lichtman SW, Pisarska K, Berman E et al, Discrepancy between self-reported and actual caloric intake and exercise in obese subjects, *N Engl J Med* (1993) **327**:1893–8.

15   Poppitt SD, Swann D, Black AE, Prentice AM, Assessment of selective under-reporting of food intake by both obese and non-obese women in a metabolic facility, *Int J Obes* (1998) **22**:303–11.

16   Holt S et al, Relationship of satiety to postprandial glycaemic, insulin and cholecystokinin responses, *Appetite* (1992) **18**:129–41.

17   Haus G, Hoerr SL, Mavis B, Robinson J, Key modifiable factors in weight maintenance: fat intake, exercise and weight cycling. *J Am Dietet Assoc* (1994) **94**:409–13.

18   Perri MG, Sears SF, Clarke JE, Towards a continuous care model of obesity management, *Diabetes Care* (1993) **16**(1):200–9.

19   Bennett GA, Behavioral therapy for obesity: a quantitative review of the effects of selected

treatment characteristics on outcome, *Behav Ther* (1986) 17:554–62.

20 American Dietetic Association, Position of the American Dietetic Association: weight management. *J Am Dietet Assoc* (1997) 97:71–4.

21 Cousins JH, Rubovits DS, Duncan JK et al, Family versus individually orientated intervention for weight loss in Mexican American Women, *Public Health Rep* (1992) 107:549–55.

22 Black DR, Threlfall WE, Partner weight status and subject weight loss: implications for cost effective programs and public health, *Addict Behav* (1989) 14:279–89,

23 Pratt CA, Development of a screening questionnaire to study attrition in weight-control programs. *Psychol Rep* (1989) 64:1007–16.

24 Barker R, Cooke B, Diet, obesity and being overweight: a qualitative research study, *Health Ed J* (1992) 51(3):117–21.

25 Brownell KD, Wadden TA, The heterogeneity of obesity: fitting treatments to individuals, *Behav Ther* (1991) 22:153–77.

26 Prentice AM, Jebb SA, Obesity in Britain: gluttony or sloth? *Br Med J* (1995) 311:437–9.

27 Lissner L, Heitmann BL, Dietary fat and obesity: evidence from epidemiology, *Eur J Clin Nutr* (1995) 49:79–90.

28 Stubbs RJ, Ritz P, Coward WA, Prentice AM, Covert manipulation of the ratio of dietary fat to carbohydrate and energy density: effect on food intake and energy balance in free-living men feeding ad libitum, *Am J Clin Nutr* (1995) 62:330–8.

29 Cotton JR, Burley VJ, Westrate JA, Blundell JE, Dietary fat and appetite: similarities and differences in the satiating effect of meals

supplemented with either fat or carbohydrate, *J Hum Nutr Dietet* (1994) 7:11–24.

30 Blundell J, Burley V, Cotton J, Lawton C, Dietary fat and the control of energy intake: evaluating the effects of fat on meal size and postmeal satiety, *Am J Clin Nutr* (1993) 57:772S–8S.

31 Stubbs RJ, Johnstone AM, Harbron CG, Reid C, Covert manipulation of energy density of high carbohydrate diets in 'pseudo free-living' humans, *Int J Obes* (1998) 22:885–92.

32 Eastwood MA, Interaction of dietary antioxidants in vivo: how fruit and vegetables prevent disease, *QJM* (1999) 92(9):527–30.

33 Collins AR, (1999) Oxidative DNA damage, antioxidants and cancer, *Bioassays* (1999) 21(3):238–46.

34 Jacob RA, Evidence that diet modification reduces in vivo oxidant damage, *Nutr Rev* (1999) 57(8):255–8.

35 DeCastro JM, Orozco S, Moderate alcohol intake and spontaneous eating patterns in humans: evidence of unregulated supplementation, *Am J Clin Nutr* (1991) 52:246–53.

36 Hill JO, Prentice AM, Sugar and body weight regulation, *Am J Clin Nutr* (1995) 62(Suppl):264S–74S.

37 Gatenby SJ, Hunt P, Rayner M, The National Food Guide: development of dietetic and nutritional characteristics, *J Hum Nutr Dietet* (1995) 8(5):47–58.

38 Hunt P, Gatenby SJ, Rayner M, A national food guide for the UK? Background and development, *J Hum Nutr Dietet* (1995) 8(5):39–46.

39 Hunt P, Gatenby SJ, Rayner M, The format for

the National Food Guide; performance and preference studies, *J Hum Nutr Dietet* (1995) 8(5):59–75.

40 Scottish Intercollegiate Guidelines Network (SIGN), *Obesity in Scotland: Integrating Prevention with Weight Management. A National Clinical Guideline Recommended for Use in Scotland by the Scottish Intercollegiate Guidelines Network* (pilot edn) (SIGN: Edinburgh, 1996).

41 James WPT, Treatment of obesity: the constraints on success. *Clin Endocr Metab* (1984) 13(3):635–59.

42 Jebb SA, Goldberg GR, Efficacy of very low-energy diets and meal replacements in the treatment of obesity, *J Hum Nutr Dietet* (1998) 11:219–25.

43 Department of Health and Social Security, *The Use of Very Low Calorie Diets in Obesity.* Report of the Working Group on Very Low Calorie Diets (HMSO: London, 1987).

44 Department of Health & Social Security, *Diet and Cardiovascular Disease.* Committee on Medical Aspects of Food Policy. Report of the Panel on Diet in Relation to Cardiovascular Disease (HMSO: London, 1984).

45 Ministry of Agriculture Fisheries and Foods, *Guidance Notes on Nutrition Labelling* (HMSO: London, 1999).

Appendix 1

Food exchange lists

Starchy foods

All of the portions below are equal to 1 starch point/exchange. Each starch point is equivalent to 80 kcal (334 kJ)

*Foods marked with * should be counted as 1 starch point or 1 fat point*

Choose . . . exchanges per day

Bread	Quantity
white/wholemeal	1 slice
bread bun/roll	$\frac{1}{2}$
chappati, no fat	1 small
crackers/crispbread	3
naan bread	*$\frac{1}{6}$th
pitta bread	1 mini or $\frac{1}{2}$ large
Cereal	
branflakes	3 tablespoons
cornflakes	3 tablespoons
muesli	2 tablespoons
porridge oats	2 tablespoons

Shreddies	3 tablespoons
Weetabix	1 bisk

Potato

oven chips	2 oz/56 g
potato, baked	1 egg size ($3\frac{1}{2}$ oz/100 g)
potato boiled	1 egg size ($3\frac{1}{2}$ oz/100 g)
cassava/plantain/yam cooked	2 oz/56 g
sweet potato	3 oz/84 g
parsnip cooked	4 oz/112 g

Rice and pasta

rice, white boiled	2 heaped tablespoons (3 oz/84 g)
rice, white raw	1 level tablespoon (1 oz/28 g)
pasta, cooked	2 heaped tablespoons (3 oz/84 g)
pasta, raw	1 level tablespoon (1 oz/28 g)

Crackers

crispbreads/crackers	3

Beans and pulses

cooked lentils, baked beans, kidney beans, chickpeas	3 oz/84 g

Fruit

All of the portions below are equal to 1 fruit exchange/point. Each fruit point is equivalent to 60 kcal/251 kJ

Choose . . . fruit exchanges per day

Fruit	Quantity
apples, oranges, pears	1 fruit
banana	1 small fruit
plums	2 large fruit
clementines/satsumas/tangerines	2 large
dates/figs	2
grapes	20

grapefruit	1
kiwi	2
mango	$\frac{3}{4}$ fruit
melon	8 oz slice
peaches	2
pineapple	2 slices (5 oz/140 g)
strawberries	6 oz/168 g
avocado	$\frac{1}{4}$ fruit (1 oz/28 g)
fresh fruit salad	2–3 tablespoons
stewed or tinned fruit	2–3 tablespoons
fruit juice, unsweetened	1 small glass (4 fl oz/120 ml)
dried fruit (raisins, currants)	1 tablespoon (1 oz/28 g)

Vegetables

All of the portions below are equal to 1 vegetable exchange/point

Choose . . . vegetable exchanges/points per day

Vegetable	Quantity
any raw, cooked, frozen, tinned vegetable	$\frac{1}{2}$ cup cooked/1 cup raw
salad	1 dessertspoon

Meat, fish and alternatives

All of the portions below are equal to 1 meat/fish/alternative point/exchange. Each meat point is equivalent to approximately 55 kcal (230 kJ)

Foods marked with * should be counted as 1 meat point <u>and 1 fat point</u>

Choose . . . exchanges per day

Meats	Quantity (cooked weights)
beef, lamb, pork, chicken, turkey (lean, fat and skin removed)	1 thin slice (1 oz/28 g)

thin sausage, grilled	*1 small (20 g)
back bacon, trimmed and grilled	*1 rasher

Offal

kidney, liver	1 tablespoon (1 oz/28 g)

Fish

cod, haddock, plaice	1 small fillet (2 oz/56 g)
herring, kipper	$\frac{1}{3}$ small fillet (1 oz/28 g)
tinned salmon, sardines, tuna (in brine or tomato sauce)	1 tablespoon
crab, prawns	2 oz/56 g
smoked salmon	1 oz/28 g

Eggs   1

Cheese

cottage	1 heaped tablespoon (2 oz/56 g)
hard cheddar type	*$\frac{1}{2}$ oz/14 g
soft brie type	*1 oz/28 g
reduced fat, hard	*1 oz/28 g

Milk and dairy foods

All of the portions below are equal to 1 milk point/exchange. Each milk point is equivalent to approximately 90 kcal (376 kJ)

Choose . . . exchanges per day

Milk	**Quantity**	
whole	$\frac{1}{4}$ pint	150 ml
semi-skimmed	$\frac{1}{3}$ pint	200 ml
skimmed	$\frac{1}{2}$ pint	300 ml

Yoghurt		
low-calorie	150 g	1 small carton
low-fat plain	150 g	1 small carton

Fats

All of the portions below are equal to 1 fat point/exchange. Each fat point is equivalent to approximately 45 kcal (188 kJ)

Choose . . . exchanges per day

Spreads	Quantity
butter, peanut butter	1 teaspoon
margarine	1 teaspoon
low fat spread (40% fat)	1 teaspoons
very low fat spread (23% fat)	2 teaspoons
All oils	1 teaspoon
Olives	18

Salad dressings	
coleslaw	2 tablespoons
mayonnaise	1 teaspoon
low-fat mayonnaise	2 teaspoons
salad cream	1 tablespoon
reduced-calorie salad cream	2 tablespoons
fat-free	4 tablespoons

Nuts	
almonds	7 whole nuts
brazils, walnuts	3 whole nuts
peanuts	16

Free foods

These foods are so low in calories that they can be taken freely

No-added-sugar squashes
Diet fizzy drinks
Sugar-free chewing gum
Tea, coffee and herbal teas

Still and fizzy mineral waters
Herbs, spices
1 tablespoon tomato ketchup, brown sauce
Vinegar
Worcester sauce
Tabasco sauce
Artificial sweeteners

Behavior therapy

John P Foreyt and Antonia A Paschali

8

Behavior therapy is now considered to be among the most widely used approaches for losing and maintaining weight.[1] The behavioral approach was originally based on psychological learning theories developed mainly by Skinner[2] and Bandura.[3] The theories suggested that behaviors were primarily learned through classical and instrumental conditioning. Conditioning strategies could therefore be used to help learn new behaviors, unlearn old ones, and modify unhealthy ones. The focus of behavior therapy has also been on behavior change per se and the modification of the environmental factors which controlled it.[4]

Behavior therapy was first applied to the treatment of obesity in the 1960s described in an article entitled 'The control of eating' published by Ferster and colleagues in a journal which went out of print after its first year of publication.[5] Ferster's work was influenced by the general principles of self-control outlined earlier by Skinner,[6] who suggested that individuals have control over their behavior through manipulation of the variables that have known influence. This viewpoint was reiterated by Goldiamond,[7] who defined the relationship between behavior (B) and environmental factors (x) as $B = f(x)$, suggesting that an individual's capability to influence known environmental factors (*x*) allowed ultimate control of his or her behaviors (*B*). Ferster et al operationalized the self-control paradigm as an integral component of a program to control overeating.[5] They suggested that the obese eat in a large variety of environmental circumstances (for example, watching television, driving in a car, lying in bed, etc), which were thought to serve as powerful cues to promote the desire and the tendency to overeat. The treatment was to reduce these cues, or stimuli, associated with the act of overeating such as by limiting all eating behavior to one location (for example sitting down at the dining room table with the television turned off).

The most successful early behavioral weight loss intervention was published by Stuart,[8] who reported that the eight obese women he treated lost an average of 17 kg at the end of 12 months. Stuart's outstanding results were the impetus for an outpouring of research interest in the use of behavioral strategies in the treatment of obesity.

During the 1970s, an impressive number of research studies were reported on the use of behavioral strategies with overweight patients. The studies typically involved 8 to 10 weeks of group treatment with mildly overweight individuals, often conducted in university settings by students completing theses or dissertations. Later patients became heavier, interventions longer, and treatment strategies

more complex. Nutrition and physical activity began to take more of a central role. Follow-ups became more common.

In the 1980s, the role of cognition became popular in behavior therapy and began to exert a major influence in behavioral interventions.[9] These cognitive-behavioral approaches focused on the identification and modification of inappropriate thought patterns and expectations associated with being overweight. For example, many obese individuals set unrealistic goals for themselves with respect to how much weight they think they can lose. When these goals are not met, they may become discouraged and lose their resolve. Realistic goal setting is used to help patients modify their expectations.

Throughout the 1990s, behavior therapy became an integral part of essentially all weight control treatment programs. Intervention typically involves a package of strategies aimed at helping patients adhere to a sensible eating plan and a realistic physical activity program. Within the overall package, the behavioral strategies are individualized based on the specific needs of the individual.[10] No single strategy or particular combination of strategies has shown itself to be superior to any other. Therefore several strategies aimed at changing inappropriate eating and increasing physical activity are presented to patients. The interventions are usually taught in groups because of cost considerations and for the support that the group members can provide to each other. However, the interventions can also be taught on an individual basis, either with a behavioral counselor or through self-help manuals.[10]

Today, a great many randomized controlled outcome studies of behavior therapy have been published.[11] They consistently show the superiority of the approach over simple dietary treatment. However, the enthusiasm of the early days of behavior modification has been supplanted by a more sober evaluation of its use because of the discouraging results of longer-term follow-up data.[10] Despite the more modest follow-up data, behavioral therapy has offered the most consistent beneficial results (apart from surgical treatments) for overweight patients and represents the gold standard of current approaches to the treatment of this refractory disease.

Description of current cognitive-behavior therapy programs

Obesity interventions that incorporate cognitive-behavioral strategies are effective in helping patients lose modest amounts of weight. Cognitive-behavior therapy (CBT) interventions last about 18 weeks. Average weight losses are about 9 kg. Attrition rates are generally low, usually less than 18%. Patients maintain about two-thirds of their losses on average at 1-year follow-up, but without

Table 8.1
Cognitive-behavioral strategies.

- *Self-monitoring*
- *Stimulus control*
- *Goal setting*
- *Problem solving*
- *Cognitive restructuring*
- *Self-rewards*
- *Relapse prevention*
- *Stress management*
- *Social support*

continued treatment gradually gain back all of their lost weight over 3 to 5 years.[12] Only a continual care model of treatment has been shown to be effective long term.[12]

Current CBT interventions typically include a number of strategies to help patients adhere to a dietary regimen and a physical activity program. These strategies include self-monitoring, stimulus control, goal setting, problem solving, cognitive restructuring, self-rewards, relapse prevention, stress management, and social support (Table 8.1).

Self-monitoring

If a physician chooses to utilize just one behavioral strategy, we recommend self-monitoring. Self-monitoring is the most important of all behavioral interventions. It involves self-observation, self-recording, and feedback of relevant behaviors by the patient. The purpose of self-monitoring is to raise the patient's awareness of eating and physical activity behaviors and the factors contributing to them. It includes the use of a food diary in which the patient writes down all foods eaten and the conditions or situations in which the eating occurred. The diary can be a simple, inexpensive notebook. The recording ideally should be done as soon as possible after the food is eaten (even better, before the food is eaten because that involves planning and structure). The feedback can include looking up and recording the number of calories or fat grams that each food contained. The patient should do the recording and the feedback, followed by reinforcement from the physician or behavioral counselor. In addition to recording food consumed, other behavioral patterns to write down might include time of day the food was eaten, where the food was eaten, mood state, and who else was present. The physician or behavioral counselor can then look at the diary and help identify patterns that might need to be changed. For example, common patterns include binge eating, night eating, or eating under stress, when tense, or bored.

Physical activity can be recorded in the same diary. Minutes of activity, along with time of day, are usually best to record. The physician can help reward consistency, trying to build a habit of daily brisk walking.

Weight should be recorded on a regular basis. We find that the more frequently the patients weigh themselves, the better the results. We recommend daily weighing at the same time each day, although we recognize that weight fluctuations are common and we make sure to discuss these issues with our patients.

Patients hate self-monitoring. When forced to do so, they under-report their intake by about a third, and over-report their physical activity by about a half. It does not matter. We believe that the primary function of self-monitoring is raising awareness of relevant behaviors, not accuracy. If physicians can motivate their patients to record their food, physical activity and weight, chances are the patients will be successful. One of our patients, 'Mary Kay', lost 28 kg and credited her success with keeping a food diary. Research has demonstrated consistently that self-monitoring is associated with improved treatment outcomes (Table 8.2).

Stimulus control

If a physician chooses to utilize two behavioral strategies, stimulus control would be the second most important one to consider.

Table 8.2
Self-monitoring.

> *Observe, record, provide feedback:*
> - *Food diary*
> - *Physical activity diary*
> - *Weight record*

Stimulus control involves identifying and modifying the environmental cues or barriers that are associated with the patient's overeating and underactivity. By changing the cues, the patient may be more likely to be successful in managing eating and physical activity. Controlling these cues ('stimulus control') may help the patient long term because their exposure is frequently related to relapse. There are probably hundreds of stimulus control strategies. It is important for the physician and patient to work together to develop practical, tailored strategies that target the patient's major difficulties. For example, some of our patients seem out of control in their eating. They eat their breakfast in the car driving to work in the morning, their lunch at their desk, and their dinner in front of the television set. They later snack in bed. Limiting their at-home eating to the kitchen table, sitting down, with the television turned off might be helpful, at least at the beginning of a program, to raise awareness of the food being eaten.

One of the most difficult problems we face with patients is helping them find the time and the motivation to be more physically active. Reviewing with them the countless benefits of physical activity, helping them reprioritize their day, and starting slowly can all be helpful. Asking patients to lay out their exercise clothes and shoes the night before as a reminder to walk or jog in the morning is a stimulus control strategy that can make it

Table 8.3
Stimulus control.

Identify and modify environmental barriers:
* Normalize eating pattern
* Lay out exercise clothes
* Find new ways to be active

easier to get moving. One study prompted patients to be more active by weekly phone calls, which significantly improved compliance to a walking program.[13]

We think that starting with one or two stimulus control strategies is easier and more sensible than asking patients to take on too many challenges all at once. We typically start with strategies to encourage patients to be more active (Table 8.3).

Goal setting

Goals for losing weight often differ between the patient and physician. We had a patient, 'Jim' who weighed 360 pounds. When we asked him what he wanted to weigh, he replied 'I just want to get down to 170 pounds'. Our response was 'Great, but let's begin by losing 30 pounds over the next 6 months'. Helping 'Jim' refocus his goals made it easier for him to lose 30 pounds over 24 weeks. Realistic goal setting, involving separating short-term goals from long-term goals, is important in preventing discouragement in the patient. Most patients will lose about 10% of their prescribing body weight in a behavioral weight loss program. Many want to lose much more than that. Focusing on short-term goals and reinforcing small positive behavioral changes can go a long way toward helping patients recognize their achievements. Short-term goals are always easier to achieve than long-term ones and give a good feeling of mastery to the patient. Focusing on the many health benefits that accrue with even modest weight losses is one way to reinforce changes (Table 8.4).

Problem solving

Losing weight involves having to learn to manage emotional issues and social events. Problem solving involves identifying and managing these situations.[9,14,15] Learning an effective approach for handling an anxious moment may involve examining a number of solutions, choosing the best one, implementing the strategy, and evaluating the outcome. For example, some patients who

have structured their eating by limiting their calories and fat grams become anxious when invited to an unfamiliar restaurant. Calling the restaurant manager ahead of time and asking for low-fat suggestions can be an effective problem-solving approach. Patients who are invited to social events where high-fat foods are going to be served can either throw up their hands in defeat or use problem solving to help them figure out strategies, like bringing a low-fat dish along with them, to stay in control. We have found that helping patients learn to deal with emotional issues and social situations is crucial to successful long-term weight management (Table 8.5).

Cognitive restructuring

Cognitive restructuring involves helping patients change their inaccurate beliefs about weight loss. For example, some patients believe that their lives will change dramatically when they lose weight. They think that they will be more loved and more successful, that

Table 8.4
Goal setting.

- *Realistic goals (10% of initial weight)*
- *Separate short-term from long-term goals*
- *Focus on health benefits*

Table 8.5
Problem solving.

Handling emotional issues and social events:
- *Examine solutions*
- *Choose one*
- *Implement strategy*
- *Evaluate outcome*

all their problems will magically disappear, and that they will be happy and content. When some of these patients do lose weight and what they thought would happen does not, they become discouraged and their motivation wanes. Cognitive restructuring encourages patients to examine their thoughts and feelings about themselves with respect to their obesity. It challenges them to change the ones that are inaccurate. Their lives may not change significantly when they lose weight. It is important to help patients understand why it is important to lose weight, such as for better health, than for unrealistic reasons.

Some patients who have been obese all their lives have trouble seeing themselves leaner, resulting in increased risk of failure because of distorted self-images. The physician can help patients identify self-defeating thoughts and change them to more productive ones. We have found that positive self-affirmations can work wonders with some patients. Having patients write down and read positive statements about themselves, such as 'I'm too sexy to be fat,' or 'I'm too good looking to be fat' can remind patients to focus on positive behavior change. Specific affirmations like 'I will walk at least 45 minutes today' and 'I will eat at least five fruit and vegetables today' can also help (Table 8.6).

Table 8.6
Cognitive restructuring.

> Changing inaccurate beliefs about weight loss:
> * Examine thoughts and feelings
> * Challenge inaccurate ones
> * Use positive self-affirmations

Self-rewards

Weight loss programs incorporating behavioral contracting have resulted in greater weight losses and lower attrition rates than programs not including these elements.[16,17] There are a number of contracting strategies that we have used with patients during weight loss interventions. The physician and patient can sign a formal contract, with the patient agreeing to make specific behavioral changes, such as walking 30 minutes a day at least three times a week over the next month. We find that it is best to begin with one or two fairly easy behaviors, like agreeing to cut down on evening snacks or to walk for a short time each day. The contract can then be updated with each meeting of patient and physician. With group interventions, small prizes or lottery draws can be used to increase motivation, interest, and help make the process of behavior change less onerous and daunting. Patients can learn to self-reward themselves for change. Individuals who self-reward themselves for achievement of behavioral goals are more likely to maintain their weight losses at 1-year follow-up than those who do not.[18,19]

In our research studies, we frequently use a refundable deposit to increase attendance at group sessions. Patients are asked to deposit a modest amount of money at the beginning of the intervention and receive it back when they attend a majority of the sessions and the measurement visits. Attrition is greatly reduced with the use of a refundable deposit. Money not returned is usually donated to a charity, such as the American Heart Association (Table 8.7).

Relapse prevention

Emotional states and social situations are major causes of relapse.[20] We teach patients to prepare for such situations. Lapses are normal. Patients need to recognize and anticipate the situations in which they might occur. Stress and anxiety, including work deadlines and taking on too many tasks, frequently get in the way of planned eating. Traveling, eating in restaurants, and attending parties make the patient vulnerable to lapses. We try to help patients recognize common situations that may lead them astray and have them design strategies to minimize the damage. If patients can predict a high-risk situation, they can usually prevent it from hurting them. Didactic training, modeling, role playing, and visualization activities (having the patients first visualize the high-risk situation and handle it successfully in imagery before actually taking part in it) can all help patients develop coping strategies to manage lapses and prevent full relapses[4] (Table 8.8).

Stress management

Stress is one of the primary predictors of losing control over eating, so learning to manage stress is critical.[21] Stress reduction strategies include diaphragmatic breathing, progressive muscle relaxation, meditation, and desensitization.[22,23] The purpose of these strategies is to reduce sympathetic nervous

Table 8.7
Self-rewards.

Using contracts for behavioral changes:
- Physician–patient contract
- Self-contract
- Refundable deposit

Table 8.8
Relapse prevention.

Preventing lapses from becoming relapses:
- Identify high-risk situations
- Didactic training
- Modeling
- Role playing
- Visualization activities

system arousal and to provide a temporary 'time-out' or distraction from the stressful event. For example, in a study investigating stress reduction, subjects were taught to use a deconditioning strategy to reduce the anxiety associated with 'eating less'. They lost significant weight (7.5% over 11.5 months), compared to subjects who were instructed to follow a balanced 1000 calorie diet without the deconditioning (they gained 6.5% over the same time period).[24] Another study trained patients in desensitization to lessen their anxiety to dieting compared to patients who were given relaxation training. The patients who learned desensitization lost more weight than those who just received the relaxation training.[25]

One of our obese Mexican–American patients, 'Rosa', attended a dinner-dance at a local community center. She told us later that she spied a German chocolate cake, her favorite, on the dinner table, but before eating any of the cake she hurried to the women's restroom and practiced her stress reduction progressive relaxation technique (muscle tensing and relaxing) that we had taught her. She told us that she became so relaxed that she 'staggered' over to the dinner table, was not at all tempted by the cake, did not eat anything at all, and danced the night away with her husband. If patients are taught strategies that they believe will help them with their food cravings, they can successfully reduce their occurrences of unwanted binging.

Stress management strategies become even more important as individuals move from weight loss phase to the weight maintenance phase.[1] In a study comparing weight maintainers to regainers, the researchers reported that both groups had a similar number of stressful events; however, the two groups differed in how they responded to the stressors. The maintainers used problem-solving skills, including stress management, or confrontive ways of coping with the stressors, compared to the relapsers who used emotion-focused or escape-avoidance strategies, such as eating, sleeping, or just wishing or hoping that the problem would go away[21] (Table 8.9).

Social support

Patients with high levels of social support are more successful at weight loss and maintenance than those without strong support systems.[17,20,26] Family members, good friends, participation in community-based programs and adult education programs at

Table 8.9
Stress management.

Stress is a primary predictor of loss of control:
• Diaphragmatic breathing
• Progressive muscle relaxation
• Meditation
• Desensitization

local colleges, or involvement in outside social activities, can serve as support networks. Peer support may be particularly useful because it may help patients manage stressful work or family-related situations, and learn to become more self-accepting. We ask our patients to take an adult interest class from a local college just to get involved with others.

Although involvement of family members in weight loss efforts has received mixed support in research studies, a review of couples' obesity treatment programs found that they were more effective in weight loss than subject-alone programs.[27] The mere presence of a spouse or family member does not guarantee success. One study found that patients whose spouses attended weight loss sessions and were trained in specific behavioral strategies such as self-monitoring lost more weight than patients whose spouses were less cooperative.[27] Interestingly, women seem to benefit more than men from weight loss programs that include spouses.[28] We think that including spouses and family members in weight loss programs is a mixed blessing.

Table 8.10
Social support.

> *Strong support systems increase weight loss and maintenance:*
> * *Family*
> * *Peer*
> * *Community*

When you can get them to cooperate, your chances of success increase. When you can not, other support networks may help (Table 8.10).

Weight loss maintenance: predictors of long-term success

Maintenance of weight loss represents the Achilles' heel of all treatment programs. Cognitive-behavioral approaches have not fared better than nonbehavioral programs over the long term. In most CBT programs, patients gradually regain their lost weight over 3 to 5 years posttreatment.[29–34] Only the continuous care model of obesity, which views obesity as a chronic disease requiring long-term intervention, has shown some success at maintenance of weight loss.[35] Continued contact by telephone, mail, or clinic visits improved maintenance in patients who had lost about 10% of initial weight during treatment.[35,36]

Physical activity is the strongest behavioral predictor of weight maintenance. Patients who exercise at home appear to do better at maintenance than those who attend health clubs.[37,38] Likewise, patients who increase their lifestyle activity, such as using stairs rather than elevators or walking rather than driving, do as well in managing weight and improving cardiovascular fitness as patients who engage in more structured exercise programs.[39,40]

Obese patients who lose significant amounts of weight will likely need to expend about 2000 to 3000 kcal per week through diet and exercise to maintain their losses.[39,41,42] For example, patients in the National Weight Control Registry who had lost at least 14 kg and maintained those losses for at least 1 year reported that they were expending an average of 2800 kcal/week to maintain their losses.[43] Although these data are discouraging for patients and illustrate the enormous difficulties faced in maintaining losses, we try to communicate to our patients that any physical activity is better than none, and we encourage patients to be more active for the health benefits that accrue, not just the weight changes.[44,45]

Additional predictors of maintenance include adherence to a low-fat eating pattern, a good support network, and a positive coping style, including the use of cognitive restructuring and stress management techniques (Table 8.11 and 8.12).

Currently, greater emphasis is being placed on broader definitions of success rather than just body weight. More importance is being placed on improvements in metabolic profiles, including lipids and glucose, self-esteem, positive body image, self-efficacy, quality of life, and improved functional capacity.[46,47] Rather than emphasizing just weight loss, behavioral clinicians are focusing on the maladaptive thoughts, negative emotions, and poor body image often associated with obesity

and highlighting the importance of helping patients accept themselves and resolving emotional issues related to eating and exercise that may be hindering long-term change[20,48,49] (Table 8.13).

Table 8.11
Weight maintenance.

- Physical activity
- Low-fat eating pattern
- Support system
- Positive coping style

Table 8.12
Improving success.

Build coping strategies for managing:
- Emotional issues
- Social events

Reinforce:
- Regular physical activity
- Problem solving
- Social support

Table 8.13
Realistic management goals.

- 10% weight loss
- Health, energy and physical activity
- Well-being and self-esteem
- Positive body image
- Accepting self

Future considerations in the management of obesity

Obesity is increasingly being seen as a chronic disease for which there is no cure. Its management requires continual care and eternal vigilance.[50] To date, intervention strategies (except for obesity surgery) have resulted in modest short-term losses, large variability, and limited clinical significance. Long-term maintenance of losses is rare. Because of the poor outcome data, long-term pharmacotherapy may have an increasingly important role in the management of obesity. Two long-term medications, orlistat and sibutramine, have been approved by the Food and Drug Administration for weight loss in the United States. Both of them result in about the same average losses during treatment as behavioral interventions, an average of 10% loss from baseline (Chapter 10). Medications may play an important role in helping patients maintain their initial treatment losses. The most effective combination of behavioral therapy and pharmacotherapy has yet to be determined.

Few intervention programs have been aimed at the treatment of obesity in children and adolescents. Given the alarming increase in the prevalence of the disease in both groups, attempts to stem this most serious public health problem are needed.

Prevention of further weight gain has likewise received little research attention.

Whether or not any public health approaches can be successful in either preventing or managing obesity remains to be seen. We believe that it is the number one public health problem in the world today. Without innovative public health approaches, the prevalence of obesity and its related health care costs can be expected to continue to increase worldwide.

References

1 King TK, Lloyd EE, Clark MM, Behavioral approaches to enhancing weight loss and maintenance. In: Rippe JM, ed, *Lifestyle Medicine* (Blackwell Science: Malden, 1999) 531–7.

2 Skinner BF, *The Behavior of Organisms: An Experimental Analysis* (Appleton-Century-Crofts: New York, 1938).

3 Bandura A, *Social Learning Theory* (Prentice-Hall: Englewood Cliffs, 1977).

4 Wing RR, Behavioral approaches to the treatment of obesity. In: Bray GA, Bouchard C, James WPT, eds, *Handbook of Obesity* (Marcel Dekker: New York, 1998) 855–73.

5 Ferster C, Nurnberger J, Levitt E, The control of eating, *J Mathetics* (1962) **1**:87–109.

6 Skinner B, *Science and Human Behavior* (Macmillan: New York, 1953).

7 Goldiamond I, Self control procedures in personal behavior problems, *Psychol Rep* (1965) **17**:851–68.

8 Stuart R, Behavioral control of overeating, *Behav Res Ther* (1967) **5**:357–65.

9 Foreyt JP, Poston WSC, What is the role of

cognitive-behavior therapy in patient management? *Obes Res* (1998) **6**:18S–22S.

10 Foreyt JP, Poston WSC, The challenge of diet, exercise and lifestyle modification in the management of the obese diabetic patient, *Int J Obes Relat Metab Disord* (1999) **23**:S5–11.

11 Wardle J, Rapoport L, Cognitive-behavioural treatment of obesity. In: Kopelman PG, Stock MJ, eds, *Clinical Obesity* (Blackwell Science: Oxford, 1998) 409–28.

12 National Institutes of Health (NIH), *Clinical Guidelines on the Identification, Evaluation, and Treatment of Overweight and Obesity: The Evidence Report* (US Government Printing Office: Washington, DC, 1998).

13 Lombard D, Lombard T, Winett R, Walking to meet health guidelines: the effects of prompting frequency and prompting structure, *Health Psychol* (1995) **14**:164–70.

14 Foreyt JP, Poston WSC, The role of the behavioral counselor in obesity treatment, *J Am Diet Assoc* (1998) **98**:S27–30.

15 Goodrick GK, Poston WSC, Kimball KT et al, Non-dieting vs. dieting treatment for overweight binge-eating women, *J Consult Clin Psychol* (1998) **66**:363–8.

16 Mavis B, Stoffelmayr B, Multidimensional evaluation of monetary incentive strategies for weight control, *Psychol Rec* (1994) **44**:239–52.

17 Foreyt JP, Goodrick GK, Factors common to successful therapy for the obese patient, *Med Sci Sports Exerc* (1991) **23**:292–7.

18 Brownell KD, Kramer FM, Behavioral management of obesity, *Med Clin North Am* (1989) **73**:185–201.

19 Kramer F, Jeffery R, Snell M, Maintenance of successful weight loss over 1 year: effects of financial contracts for weight maintenance or

participation in skill training, *Behav Ther* (1986) **17**:295–301.

20 Foreyt JP, Goodrick GK, *Living without Dieting* (Warner Books: New York, 1994).

21 Kayman S, Bruvold W, Stern JS, Maintenance and relapse after weight loss in women: behavioral aspects, *Am J Clin Nutr* (1990) **52**:800–7.

22 Everly G, *A Clinical Guide to the Treatment of the Human Stress Response* (Plenum Press: New York, 1990).

23 Lichstein KL, *Clinical Relaxation Strategies* (John Wiley: New York, 1988).

24 Nagler W, Androff A, Investigating the impact of deconditioning anxiety on weight loss, *Psychol Rep* (1990) **66**:595–600.

25 Pietre AJ, Nicki RM, Desensitization of dietary restraint anxiety and its relationship to weight loss, *J Behav Ther Exp Psychiatry* (1994) **25**:153–4.

26 Stunkard AJ, Wadden TA, Psychological aspects of severe obesity, *Am J Clin Nutr* (1992) **55**:524S–32S.

27 Brownell KD, Heckerman CL, Westlake RJ et al, The effect of couples training and partner cooperativeness in the behavioral treatment of obesity, *Behav Res Ther* (1978) **16**:323–33.

28 Wing RR, Marcus M, Epstein L, Jawad A, A 'family-based' approach to the treatment of obese type II diabetic patients, *J Consult Clin Psychol* (1991) **59**:156–62.

29 Perri MG, Fuller PR, Success and failure in the treatment of obesity: where do we go from here? *Med Exerc Nutr Health* (1995) **4**:255–72.

30 Foreyt J, Goodrick GK, Evidence for success of behavior modification in weight loss and control, *Ann Intern Med* (1993) **119**:698–701.

31 Kramer F, Jeffery R, Forster J, Snell M, Long-

term follow-up of behavioral treatment for obesity: patterns of weight regain in men and women, *Int J Obes* (1989) **13**:123–36.

32 Safer DJ, Diet, behavior modification, and exercise: a review of obesity treatments from a long-term perspective, *South Med J* (1991) **84**:1470–4.

33 Stalonas PM, Perri MG, Kerzner AB, Do behavioral treatments of obesity last? A five-year follow-up investigation, *Addict Behav* (1984) **9**:175–83.

34 Wadden TA, Sternberg JA, Letizia KA et al, Treatment of obesity by very low calorie diet, behavior therapy, and their combination: a five-year perspective, *Int J Obes* (1989) **13**:39–46.

35 Perri M, Nezu A, Viegener B, *Improving the Long-term Management of Obesity: Theory, Research, and Clinical Guidelines* (John Wiley: New York, 1992).

36 Perri MG, McAllister DA, Gange JJ et al, Effects of four maintenance programs on the long-term management of obesity. *J Consult Clin Psychol* (1988) **56**:529–34.

37 King AC, Haskell WL, Young DR et al, Long-term effects of varying intensities and formats of physical activity on participation rates, fitness and lipoproteins in men and women aged 50–60 years, *Circulation* (1995) **91**:2596–604.

38 Perri MG, Martin AD, Leermakers EA, Sears SF, Effects of group versus home-based exercise training in healthy older men and women, *J Consult Clin Psychol* (1997) **65**:278–85.

39 Anderson D, Wadden TA, Treating the obese patient, *Arch Fam Med* (1999) **8**:156–67.

40 Dunn AL, Marcus BH, Kampert JB et al, Comparison of lifestyle and structured interventions to increase physical activity and cardiorespiratory fitness: a randomized trial, *JAMA* (1999) **281**:327–34.

41 Jakicic JM, Winters C, Lang W, Wing RR, Effects of intermittent exercise and use of home exercise equipment on adherence, weight loss, and fitness in overweight women: a randomized trial, *JAMA* (1999) **282**:1554–60.

42 Jakicic JM, Polley BA, Wing RR, Accuracy of self-reported exercise and the relationship with weight loss in overweight women, *Med Sci Sports Exerc* (1998) **30**:634–8.

43 Klem ML, Wing RR, McGuire MT et al, A descriptive study of individuals successful at long-term maintenance of substantial weight loss, *Am J Clin Nutr* (1997) **66**:239–46.

44 Blair SN, Kohl HW, Paffenbarger RS et al, Physical fitness and all-cause mortality: a prospective study of healthy men and women, *JAMA* (1989) **262**:2395–401.

45 Blair SN, *Living with Exercise* (American Health Publishing Company: Dallas, 1991).

46 Foster GD, Wadden TA, Vogt RA et al, What is a reasonable weight loss? Patients' expectations and evaluations of obesity treatment outcomes, *J Consult Clin Psychol* (1997) **65**:79–85.

47 Wilson GT, Behavioral treatment of obesity: thirty years and counting, *Adv Behav Res Ther* (1994) **16**:31–75.

48 Ciliska D, *Beyond Dieting: Psychoeducational Interventions for Chronically Obese Women: A Non-dieting Approach* (Brunner/Mazel: New York, 1990).

49 Polivy J, Herman CP, Undieting: a program to help people stop dieting, *Int J Eat Disord* (1992) **11**:261–8.

50 Foreyt J, Pendleton V, Management of obesity, *Prim Care Rep* (2000) **6**:20–30.

The physical activity approach to the treatment of overweight and obesity

Kenneth R Fox and Angie Page

9

Introduction

When the growing problem of overweight and obesity is mentioned, the issues that immediately spring to mind for most people will be food intake and overeating. Until the last 5 years, lack of physical activity has received at best secondary attention. Attributions to gluttony rather than sloth appears to be characteristic of not only the general public, but also health professionals and policy makers. General practitioners and practice nurses are much more likely to refer overweight and obese patients to dietitians rather than exercise specialists. Even today, almost all commercially-driven weight loss programmes focus primarily on dieting, with only cursory interest in exercise as a means of weight control.

The limited credence given to inactivity as a cause of obesity and overweight is not entirely clear. Research evidence supporting the role of exercise in health improvement, weight loss and the prevention of weight gain has only emerged in the past 10 years or so and is still gathering pace. In the meantime, the general public have taken the view that exercise does little for weight loss or that its effects are too slow in comparison to dieting to be of benefit. Many health professionals perhaps believe that achieving exercise adoption and compliance in obese people is futile because of their low levels of motivation.

This chapter aims to summarize the growing evidence base for the role of exercise in the treatment and prevention of overweight and obesity. A broad perspective of treatment that takes into account health risk, long-term weight management, psychological well-being and motivation for behaviour change is adopted. This is translated into recommendations for physical activity promotion for weight management in different lifespan populations.

Throughout the chapter the terms 'physical activity' and 'exercise' are used. Physical activity has the broader meaning of the two and encapsulates all significant bodily movement engaged in through the daily routine such as housework, walking and cycling as a form of transport, shopping and active hobbies. Exercise is confined to those physical activities (which might include some from this list) that are undertaken with the intention of improving aspects of health, fitness or weight management. Exercise is the main focus of almost all of the summarized research discussed in this chapter.

Exercise and health benefits in obesity

Typically, the merits of physical activity are presented in terms of its effectiveness in promoting weight loss. However, in recent years there has been a general shift in emphasis in obesity treatment from large weight losses to moderate weight loss and improved health or metabolic status as the key outcome. Particular emphasis has been placed on working towards healthier levels of blood pressure, blood lipids, glucose tolerance and insulin sensitivity and the role of weight loss in achieving these changes.

Throughout the last decade, evidence has accumulated to show that physical activity has a key role to play in both normal weight and obese individuals in terms of reduced risk of mortality and several diseases. Active living represents normality and it is perhaps not surprising that years of sedentary habits lead to loss of functional capacity and increased probability of serious health problems. Inactive living carries an independent 2-fold risk for all-cause mortality,[1,2] and this is similar to the risk of hypertension, hyperlipidemia, and smoking (Figure 9.1). Several major health authorities across the world are now convinced that physical inactivity should be regarded as a fourth primary risk factor for coronary heart disease and stroke.[3–5] Physical activity has additional health benefits which include reduced risk of colon cancer and improved physical fitness and psychological well-being.[6] Furthermore, those individuals who are successful in improving from low to high fitness appear to reduce their risks considerably.[7] This means

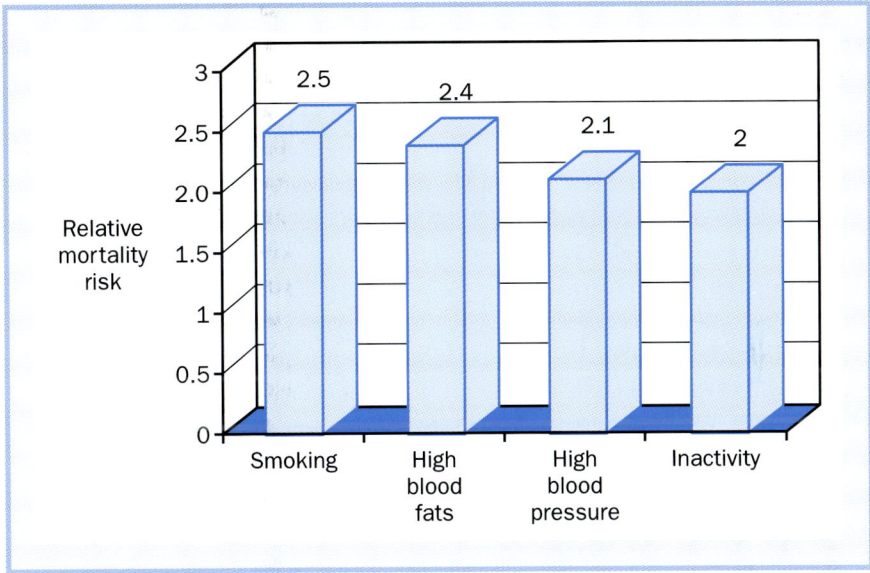

Figure 9.1
Physical inactivity: the fourth primary risk factor for coronary heart disease and stroke (Data from Powell et al[2]).

that all sedentary individuals should be encouraged to be active regardless of their weight status.

There are at least two reasons why increased physical activity may be particularly important for the health of overweight and obese individuals. First, they are more likely to be in the least active sector of the population,[8,9] and are more prone to excessive time spent in sedentary pursuits such as TV watching.[10] Second, they have a higher risk of coronary heart disease, diabetes and colon cancer, problems that physical activity may

successfully help protect against. If these two assumptions hold true, then the obese person who manages to be active should be much better off in terms of prognosis for health. Recent evidence has emerged to support this. Lee and colleagues found that those adults who are mildly obese but who have a reasonable level of cardiorespiratory fitness have a death rate about 50% of lean individuals who are unfit, even when variables such as smoking are taken into consideration.[11,12] It appears that it is highly possible to be fit and healthy even when obese, so long as it is accompanied by regular exercise.

Recently, the American College of Sports Medicine (ACSM)[13] and the US National Institutes of Health and National Heart, Lung, and Blood Institute (NIH)[14] commissioned reviews of the state of evidence for the preparation of consensus statements regarding the health benefits of physical activity for overweight and obese populations. They concluded that observational epidemiological studies had established the following:

- Overweight and obese individuals who are active and fit have lower rates of disease and death than overweight and obese individuals who are inactive and unfit.
- Overweight or obese individuals who are active and fit are less likely to develop obesity-related chronic diseases and have an early death than normal-weight persons who lead sedentary lives.
- Inactivity and low cardiorespiratory fitness are as important as overweight or obesity as predictors of mortality, at least in men.

Death rates appear to be reduced primarily through cardiovascular disease. There is also observational evidence to show that increased physical activity in obese men and women reduces the risk of colon cancer and also limits the risk of breast and endometrial cancers in obese women.[15] As yet the mechanisms for the beneficial effects of exercise in the obese have not been fully identified. Randomized controlled trials have generally failed to show that aerobic training dramatically improves the lipoprotein profile of overweight or obese men and women beyond the effects of a hypocaloric diet.[16] However, activity in obese individuals is associated with a lower incidence of hypertension and trials show that aerobic training can reduce hypertension, independent of changes in body weight, although this is no more effective than dieting.[17] A promising area, sometimes referred to as metabolic fitness, is the beneficial effects of exercise on insulin action and glucose intolerance.[18] This is clearly important in the prevention and treatment of type 2 diabetes, the incidence of which is dramatically elevated in the obese.

Less well researched is the impact of exercise on mental well-being. It has been shown to be effective in reducing clinical depression[19,20] and can also improve physical self-perceptions such as body image and physical competence.[21] These are problems which are widespread, particularly in obese women.

Clearly, if the main concern for obesity is its association with early mortality, disease and low levels of mental well-being, then physical activity promotion has to be considered a critical part of treatment.

Exercise and weight management

Exercise has several potential effects in weight management. It may result in weight and body fat losses and help individuals sustain their weight loss over the longer term. It may also help prevent weight gain across the lifespan or attenuate the degree of weight gain that is typically experienced through early and late middle age.

Exercise and weight loss

Recently several reviews, some of them meta-analytical, have addressed the research literature on the effectiveness of exercise in weight loss.[22–26] There is considerable variation in results from individual studies and rarely are the details of the exercise programme and the context in which it operates adequately described to enable full judgement. Only recent studies comply with current recommendations aimed at improving health and long-term exercise adherence and so it is difficult to judge the effectiveness of best known exercise practice. However, the general conclusions of these reviews, and in agreement with the most recent review of Wing,[27] is that randomized controlled trials have established the following:

• Exercise by itself results in modest weight loss of the order of 0.5 kg to 1 kg per month.

• Exercise and diet together provide greater weight loss than diet or exercise alone.

A typical three of four session a week aerobic exercise/walking programme would produce between 600 and 1000 kcal extra energy expenditure (depending on body weight) and this would roughly explain this degree of weight loss. Exercise is effective, particularly over the long term; however, the rate of loss is often disappointing to the patient who wishes to lose large amounts of weight rapidly. Weight loss due to exercise also seems to be less in females than in males. Furthermore, exercise for severely obese patients is usually too difficult for them to accumulate sufficient energy expenditure for significant amounts of weight loss. For this reason, exercise becomes more important as the degree of obesity diminishes, and where prevention of further weight gain rather than substantial weight loss is targeted.

This is substantiated by evidence that exercise has a differential effect on the source of weight lost. When exercise is added to a hypocaloric diet, there is a greater loss of fat mass and conservation of lean tissue (mainly muscle mass) when compared to diet alone.[22,24,27] This is likely to be important in the long term as fat-free mass largely determines resting metabolic rate, the degree of energy expended by the body while at rest, and this is the bulk of daily energy expenditure for all but highly active athletes. For this reason, resistance (weight training) exercise has recently been investigated. One study using magnetic resonance imaging indicated no loss of muscle tissue during weight loss in obese women undergoing a resistance exercise programme and diet.[28]

The effect of exercise on high-risk abdominal fat deposition, which is characteristic of men and postmenopausal women, was recently reviewed by Ross and Janssen[29] and by the US National Institutes of Health and National Heart, Lung and Blood Institute.[14] The general consensus was that exercise is effective in reducing abdominal adiposity in overweight and obese adults. This may eventually prove to be significant in terms of long-term health outcomes.

In summary, the amount of weight loss due to exercise may seem disappointing, especially as it cannot compete with dieting for rapid weight loss. However, when viewed over the longer term its effect on energy balance, both through the extra energy expended during the activity itself and through higher resting metabolic rate, is likely to be very important for weight control. It is also very important through its contribution to health and fitness gain for any person undergoing weight loss.

Exercise and maintenance of weight loss

Although weight loss in itself is difficult, keeping weight off in the long term seems to be achieved by only a small percentage and as such has to be regarded as exceptional. King and Tribble reviewed the long-term effects of programmes with follow-up measures of at least 6 months.[30] The average sustained weight loss was 4.0 kg in four diet-only programmes, 4.9 kg in five exercise-only programmes and 7.2 kg in three diet and exercise programmes. Wing reported that of the six randomized control trials using exercise, weight losses were greater in the diet and exercise versus the diet only groups at 1-year follow-up.[27] However, the differences in only two studies were significant.[31,32] A third study with only 6 months follow-up also found significantly better sustained weight loss and fat loss, and a greater resting metabolic rate in those who exercised.[33] Although the evidence from randomized controlled trials is still not strong, the effect is consistently supported by correlational data showing that physical activity levels are positively related to the amount of sustained weight loss.[27]

The reasons for this effect are still unknown. The additional energy expended through physical activity will contribute, as will any increase or maintenance of lean tissue mass over diet only groups. However, there is also the possibility that those who become successful at exercise become more positive, confident and feel in better control, with the result that they are better equipped psychologically to manage their eating more successfully. However, this remains a hypothesis that requires further research.

Exercise and prevention of weight gain

Several national surveys have shown that overweight and obese people are likely to be less active than normal weight individuals.[34,35] This effect is stronger in women than men. Similarly, a recent pan-European study indicated a graded profile of increased time spent watching television with increased BMI group.[36] In another study, using the doubly-labelled water method, Schulz and Schoeller found an association between percentage body fat and nonbasal energy expenditure of $r = -0.83$ in females and $r = -0.55$ in males.[37] While this evidence consistently shows that fatter people are more likely to be low in physical activity and higher in sedentary pursuits such as TV watching, it provides no indication of whether inactivity is a result of being overweight perhaps because it becomes less comfortable, or the cause of overweight through its effect on positive energy balance.

Prentice and Jebb have graphically demonstrated that indirect indicators of inactivity (number of cars per household and hours per week of television) have increased in parallel with the rapid growth in obesity in Britain over the past two decades.[38] The view is held that the advances in technology and availability of cheap labour-saving devices have caused subtle but widespread secular decreases in daily energy expenditure. Fewer active occupations, electrical appliances that save time and effort in the home, work and shopping environment, increasing reliance on cars for transport and the increased availability of attractive home screen entertainment have contributed to less movement and physical effort, which is having a profound effect on weight status, particularly in those individuals from families who are susceptible to weight gain. If this is the case, then public health approaches are required to promote compensatory exercise in order to redress the energy balance. This in turn would prevent, or at least attenuate, the weight gain that is typical as people approach and pass through middle age.

There is some cross-sectional evidence to support this. The US Behavior Risk Factor Surveillance System (BRFSS) study provided data on over 6000 men and 12 500 women who self-reported their exercise and sport participation.[23] When compared to the mean weights of those reporting no significant activity, those who were active through walking, running, cycling, aerobics or golf showed a lower weight with the greatest difference for activities of higher energy expenditure. All differences were independent of height, race, education, smoking and energy intake restriction.

Several large-sample, prospective observational studies, with six providing at least 5-year follow-up data, have investigated the effect of activity habits on subsequent weight gain/loss. Although the findings are variable among these studies, the overall conclusion of recent reviews is that activity and increasing activity at least attenuate weight gain in the population.[9,10] The risk of significant weight gain is reduced substantially in several studies. For example, in the NHANES study of Williamson et al, men who reported low activity at baseline and follow-up were 3.9 times more likely to gain 8–13 kg over the 10-year period than men who reported high activity on both occasions.[39] The risk of very high weight gain (>13 kg) for women was also high for those who reported low activity on both occasions, although confidence intervals were wide. DiPietro and colleagues looked at the effect of cardiorespiratory fitness levels on subsequent weight status in 4599 men and 724 women over an average of 7 years.[40] Improvements in fitness over the period substantially reduced the risk of weight gain and appeared to precede it, supporting its causal role. A decrease in physical activity was associated with a risk of weight gain. In further support, a recent 2-year longitudinal study by Ching et al showed that increased physical activity and reduced TV/video watching time over the period was associated with attenuated weight gain.[41] The evidence that physical activity causes weight loss over the long term at the population level, however, is not so strong.

In summary, inactivity over several years is associated with greater amounts of weight

gain. Improving activity or cardiorespiratory fitness reduces the risk of such weight gain. Long-term activity habits therefore seem to be very important in long-term weight management. This has important possibilities for reducing the percentage of the population who eventually put on sufficient weight to be classified as clinically obese. No other lifestyle variable, such as reduced fat intake, has shown similar effects.

Physical activity recommendations

The evidence presented to this point indicates quite clearly that for the sake of improved health and long-term weight management, physical activity should be an essential part of any treatment plan for overweight or obesity. The remaining part of this chapter will focus on appropriate guidelines for exercise for adults and also for children and adolescents.

Physical activity guidelines for adults

In the 1970s, the ACSM provided guidelines for exercise for the improvement of aerobic fitness. The recommendation of aerobic exercise of three to four times per week at 60–80% of maximum heart rate for at least 20 minutes became widely accepted as a standard formula for practitioners. It is now clear that this prescription is *not* appropriate for all health contexts, and in particular is too demanding and restrictive for overweight or obese individuals. Examination of the epidemiological evidence clearly shows that the greatest gains in public health are to be made by moving the sedentary sector of the population, in which the overweight and obese are over-represented, to moderate levels of activity. The US Center for Disease Control and Prevention in collaboration with the ACSM,[42] the Health Education Authority,[5] and the Quebec Consensus Conference on Physical Activity and Health,[43] after thorough reviews of existing evidence, independently produced similar new

guidelines for activity promotion. These are more appropriate to health and also acceptable for the overweight and obese (Table 9.1).

For health, every adult, regardless of whether or not they are overweight, should aim to accumulate 30 minutes of moderate intensity physical activity equivalent to brisk walking on at least 5 days per week (see Table 9.2 for other examples). The intensity, duration and frequency of such a programme is sufficient to improve fitness[44] and provide important protection from cardiovascular diseases and all-cause mortality in those who were previously sedentary or low in activity.[45] Additionally, in the overweight and obese, it

Table 9.1
Recommendations for the appropriate amount of activity for health for adults.

Health Education Authority[5]
- *People should take 30 minutes of moderate intensity physical activity, such as a sustained brisk walk, on at least 5 days of the week*
- *Ideally these 30 minutes should be one period of sustained activity, but shorter bouts of 15 minutes, are also beneficial*

US Center for Disease Control and Prevention[42]
- *Every US adult should accumulate 30 minutes or more of moderate-intensity physical activity on most, preferably all, days of the week*

Quebec Consensus Conference[43]
For good health, physical activity should:
- *Involve large muscle groups*
- *Impose more than a customary load*
- *Require a minimum total of 700 kcal/week*
- *Be performed regularly, if possible daily*

(In practice, sustained rhythmic exercise such as brisk walking for 20 to 30 minutes would fulfil this requirement in most adults.)

Table 9.2
Examples of a healthy package of moderate physical activity.

Washing and waxing a car for 45–60 minutes	*Less vigorous, longer time*
Washing windows or floors for 45–60 minutes	
Playing volleyball for 45 minutes	
Gardening for 45–60 minutes	
Wheeling self in wheelchair for 30–40 minutes	
Walking 1.75 miles in 35 minutes	
Bicycling 5 miles in 30 minutes	
Ballroom dancing for 30 minutes	
Pushing a stroller 1.5 miles in 30 minutes	
Raking leaves for 30 minutes	
Walking 2 miles in 30 minutes	
Water aerobics for 30 minutes	
Swimming lengths for 20 minutes	
Wheelchair basketball for 20 minutes	
Rope skipping for 15 minutes	
Running 1.5 miles in 15 minutes	
Stairclimbing for 15 minutes	*More vigorous, shorter time*
(if performed daily: energy equivalent of 800–1500 kcal per week for overweight people)	

Modified from reference 3.

will increase energy expenditure above baseline by between 800 and 1500 kcal per week, dependent on body weight, which amounts to a fat equivalent of 5 to 8 kg per year.

Unlike vigorous activity, which depletes glycogen stores as a source of energy, light to moderately intense activity maximizes lipid utilization, eventually drawing fat from adipose tissue, particularly when accompanied by a low-fat diet. Furthermore, as the length of the exercise session increases, the body relies more heavily on fat as fuel. This would suggest that lighter exercise for longer duration is more effective for weight management than intense and shorter periods. However, there are also motivational considerations against which to balance the physiological effects of exercise. Prescribing exercise in short versus long bouts has been shown to increase exercise participation in overweight women during a 20-week period.[46] Recently, Jakicic and colleagues demonstrated a 'dose–response' of weight loss to exercise with the amount of weight lost significantly greater in those overweight participants who averaged at least 200 minutes per week of exercise (−13.1 kg) compared to those averaging at least 150 minutes per week (−8.5 kg) and those averaging less than 150 minutes per week (−3.5 kg) over an 18-month period.[47] These data provide strong support for the need for large volumes of exercise for sustained weight loss. How the volume is achieved through shorter or longer periods may be less important and down to individual preference.

Resistance exercise using weight machines has also been given some consideration for weight loss. The energy expenditure incurred through the physical work will be significant, but there is also the possibility that this form of exercise will maintain or even increase muscle mass, thus increasing resting metabolic rate. There are insufficient numbers of well-controlled studies to establish the effectiveness of resistance exercise at this point. However, it will improve muscular function, it will increase energy expenditure, it does appear popular with participants and therefore it would be appropriate to include it in an exercise programme for the overweight or obese.

Besides regular daily programmed exercise, for people who are overweight or obese for whom a primary consideration is creating a negative energy balance, increasing incidental movement throughout the day is also important. All movement expends energy and physical activity using large muscle groups such as the legs and arms uses most energy. Energy expended is a function of weight times distance moved and greater amounts of energy are used when moving body weight, particularly up slopes or stairs. Even though activity of low intensity, such as housework, is slower in expending energy compared to moderate or vigorous intensity activity, it is likely to occur more frequently and therefore contribute significantly over weeks and months to long-term energy balance.

Furthermore, overweight people are more likely to spend time watching television.[36] This not only takes away valuable time for energy expenditure, it is associated with the consumption of energy-dense snacks. Reductions in sedentary time may therefore be as important as increases in time spent in exercise. This suggests that professionals helping overweight and obese people become more active for health and weight loss need to suggest the following as strategies:

- A regular daily routine of walking or the equivalent
- Inclusion of sessions of resistance exercise, low impact aerobics or swimming
- More movement and physical effort throughout the day
- An active hobby such as gardening
- Reductions in time spent watching television

Exercise and food intake

There is a widespread belief among the general public that exercise does little to assist weight loss because it increases appetite and therefore offsets any extra expenditure of energy through greater energy intake. Research is showing this to be a fallacy. Blundell and King have examined the literature in depth and make several conclusions which are significant for those considering exercise as a means of weight management.[48,49] They confirm that there is at best only a weak coupling between food consumption and exercise, and this is especially the case at low levels of exercise (sedentary living). Engaging in physical activity therefore does not automatically generate an increase in the desire or drive to eat more. It is more likely that exercise for an hour or two will temporarily suppress the appetite and over the following hours or days there will be no appreciable change in the amount of food intake. If there is any drive for particular types of foods, it is likely to be for carbohydrates to replenish muscle glycogen stores. Very heavy exercise, similar to that of athletes engaging in high-level training, will stimulate compensation and increase food intake after a period of adjustment, but this is unlikely to be the case for the average person interested in weight loss. Furthermore, when an individual becomes sedentary, food intake is not likely automatically to reduce to the lower energy expenditure, therefore increasing the chances of weight gain.

There is also the belief that the energy imbalance caused by exercise is easily wiped out by the intake of energy-dense foods such as a chocolate bar. Unfortunately it is true that 30 minutes of exercise can be undermined by 30 seconds of eating!

Although there appear to be no strong physiological drives to eat more after exercise, psychosocial drives may come into play if individuals start to believe that because of their exercise they are in a position to reward themselves through eating more of their favourite foods. Research has shown us that there is a tendency to overestimate how much exercise we have accomplished and underestimate how much we have eaten, therefore to juggle intake and expenditure cognitively would appear to be a precarious strategy.

Facilitating behaviour change

As with normal-weight people, the main exercise challenge for health professionals remains the facilitation of long-term behaviour change. The Jakicic study showed that overweight individuals can achieve relatively high levels of activity per week.[47] This is supported by other studies that have shown that some overweight or obese individuals have been successful in maintaining an exercise programme of up to 18 months.[31,50,51] This is in contrast to beliefs held by many professionals that obese individuals are a lost cause, although it is true that the success rate is not high and that exercise is particularly difficult in very obese adults who often suffer joint, back and chafing problems. Overweight and obese individuals present a particularly needy but difficult case. They are less likely to be active, less susceptible to active health messages and are more likely to drop out early from formal exercise sessions than normal-weight individuals.[52] However, it is difficult to judge the quality of exercise programmes from their descriptions in the literature. Often, parameters such as frequency, duration and intensity only are reported. Over recent years, exercise psychology, using principles from behavioural and health psychology, has made it clear that there are key psychosocial and contextual elements such as the qualities of the exercise specialist, that are critical to the determination of the adherence/dropout ratio. Clearly these need to be taken into consideration if the effectiveness of programmes for overweight and obese individuals is to be maximized.

Readiness to change behaviour is a key factor in the success of weight loss programmes.[14] The limited amount of research that focuses on the psychology of exercise in the obese suggests that many have misconceptions about the type and amount of activity required that acts as an initial barrier to exercise adoption. A staged approach would suggest that exercise expectations and decision-making should be addressed initially,[53,54] perhaps using techniques found in motivational interviewing,[55] or activity counselling and contracting.[56] Furthermore, principles from cognitive behaviour therapy and behaviour therapy will be required to address exercise identity issues and to introduce behaviour change strategies. For example, social physique anxiety and low body image are pronounced, particularly in obese women, and this can pose a serious obstacle to exercise adoption and maintenance. Most will have limited experience with self-regulatory and exercise behaviour management skills such as goal setting, monitoring and cue utilization. Social support from family, friends and exercise partners is also likely to be important. It is also likely that aversion to exercise for some has meant that they have a very restricted and flawed knowledge base about exercise, and so an educational component will be required if exercise expertise and independence are to develop. In short, similar to eating and smoking, exercise is a health behaviour with sufficiently crucial implications that it requires professional support to facilitate change.

To date, the effectiveness of such a support system for enhancing long-term adherence in the obese or overweight has not been fully addressed. However, a group exercise programme specifically for overweight women that focused on peer support has reported attendance rates of over 90%.[57] Jakicic et al recently reported that providing home exercise treadmills improved long-term weight loss and fat loss due to greater maintenance of exercise behaviour during the final 6 months of treatment.[47] Anderson and Fox indicated that provision of an exercise specialist in an obesity treatment programme was able to satisfy exercise support needs and this was associated with increased exercise.[58] As with other health behaviours, long-term adherence often depends on opportunity for sustained contact.[59]

Physical activity guidelines for children and adolescents

Obesity is not restricted to adulthood. Data are sparse for trends in overweight/obesity in children, but in the USA there has been a significant increase from 4% in 6–11-year-old boys and girls in 1963–65 to 11% in boys and 10% in girls in 1990–94. Similar increases are evident for the 12–17-year-old group.[60] Figures from the UK also suggest that there is a problem of obesity in children, with recent data from a representative sample of 2630 children showing obesity rates from 10% at age 6 to 17% at age 15 years.[61] In these studies, obesity is defined as above the 95th percentile for BMI related to national age and gender reference points.[62] This level of obesity has a strong likelihood of persisting into adulthood and adding to the already burgeoning adult incidence. It is also associated with several current adverse health outcomes including hyperlipidemia, high

blood pressure and early symptoms of type 2 diabetes.[63] Effective long-term treatment options for obese children are currently limited, but Barlow and Dietz suggest that the primary goal of managing uncomplicated childhood obesity should be healthy eating and physical activity, not achievement of ideal body weight.[63]

Guidelines for health

As with adults, it is critical that children who are overweight or obese at minimum achieve the recommendations of physical activity for health for their age. Two consensus conferences held during the last decade have addressed the activity needs of young people. Achieving standard recommendations has been even more difficult than with adults. Few children show serious deterioration in their health due to low activity levels, probably because there has been insufficient time, and therefore there are no strong epidemiological endpoints on which to establish relationships. Table 9.3 shows the guidelines developed by Sallis and Patrick for adolescents.[64] These are more prescriptive than later recommendations in that they require sustained (20 minutes or more at a time), moderate to vigorous levels of exertion in three or more sessions per week. Those produced by Biddle et al,[65] on behalf of the Health Education Authority, aim for a 'volume' approach. This is in line with recommendations for physical activity in

Table 9.3
Recommendations for appropriate amount of activity for health for young people.

Sallis and Patrick[64]
- *All adolescents should be physically active daily, or nearly every day, as part of play, games, sports, work, transportation, recreation, physical education or planned exercise, in the context of the family, school, and community activities*
- *Adolescents should engage in three or more sessions per week of activities that last 20 minutes or more at a time and that require moderate to vigorous levels of exertion*

Health Education Authority[65]
- *All young people should participate in physical activity of at least moderate intensity for 1 hour per day*
- *Young people who currently undertake little activity should participate in physical activity of at least moderate intensity for at least half an hour per day*
- *At least twice per week, some of these activities should help to enhance and maintain muscular strength and flexibility and bone health*

---

obese children, where the focus is on increased energy expenditure, regardless of the way it is achieved. Children simply need to move their body weight more often and for longer periods.

Activity for weight loss

Epstein and Goldfield recently reviewed the area of physical activity in the treatment of childhood overweight and obesity.[66] They included studies lasting at least 2 months where there had been randomization or matching on demographic or anthropometric variables to different types of exercise programmes or no-exercise comparison groups. Only 13 studies were identified and variations in age, gender definitions of obesity and exercise prescriptions made conclusions

difficult. However, when comparing diet to diet plus exercise, results from six studies indicated that diet plus exercise improved short-term obesity treatment by almost half a standard deviation above and beyond the effect from diet alone. Exercise also increased fitness levels in obese children, whether compared to diet alone or to no-exercise controls.

The work of Epstein and colleagues provides some insight into the merit of lifestyle versus traditional programmed aerobic exercise when combined with dietary intervention.[67] The programmed approaches required that children achieve their activity goal through structured sessions of one activity mode. The lifestyle approach allowed children to choose how they achieved their activity goal, combining any physical activity they wished. Two further groups were given calorie-limited diets (diet/lifestyle, diet/programmed) along with their activity. Figure 9.2 shows a comparison of BMI changes for four different programmes. All groups showed a significant reduction in weight loss up to 6 months, but both the diet + programmed and programmed activity groups showed a significant increase in weight from maintenance to follow-up. The lifestyle groups maintained a greater proportion of weight loss over the time period.

Through systematic research, Epstein and colleagues have also provided evidence to support the use of exercise for long-term management of childhood obesity.[68] In one study weight change after either a lifestyle versus calisthenics exercise programmes were compared.[69] At 12 months, all groups showed similar reductions in percentage overweight, but at 10 years both the aerobic and lifestyle groups had maintained their level of overweight compared to the calisthenics group. Further work is needed, but these results would support that a more flexible approach to exercise/activity

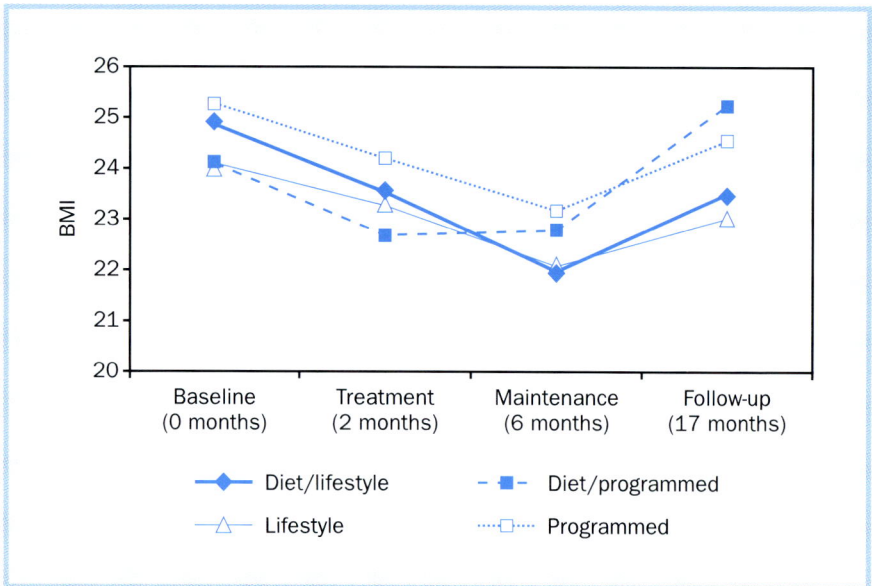

Figure 9.2
Changes in BMI over 17 months after four different exercise programmes.[67]

recommendations produces better long-term maintenance of activity and this has an effect on weight loss.

Sedentary time and obesity

As well as reinforcing physical activity behaviours, there is evidence that reducing access to sedentary behaviours can increase activity levels in obese children. To date, a stronger relationship has been detected between patterns of sedentary living (such as the amount of time spent watching television) and obesity, than physically active pursuits and obesity.[70] Recently, Gortmaker and colleagues examined longitudinal data between 1986 and 1990 on hours of TV watching and prevalence of obesity in a nationally representative sample of 746 children.[71] The odds of being overweight were 4.6 (2.2–9.6) times greater when viewing exceeded 5 hours compared with 0–2 hours per day. Additionally, the odds of developing obesity and remission from obesity were linked to time spent watching TV, with estimates of attributable risk for obesity as high as 60% linked to degree of TV watching. The conclusion of the authors is that reductions in TV time may be effective in preventing some incidence of obesity.

Robinson, in a recent innovative study, tested this idea using a randomized controlled trial featuring a school-based educational intervention.[72] The intervention, which was based on Bandura's social cognitive theory, incorporated 18 lessons of 30 to 50 minutes into the standard school curriculum taught by the usual teachers. After initial self-monitoring children were challenged to watch no television, videos or play any computer games for 10 days. After this 'turnoff' period children were encouraged to follow a 7-hour per week TV-watching 'budget', and households were provided with monitoring devices. Compared to the control group, the intervention group ($n = 106$, age 8.95 (± 0.64) years) significantly decreased by 6.5 hours, according to the childrens' self-report, and 3.5 hours, according to the parents' report. This was accompanied by small but significant relative decreases in body mass index, triceps skinfold thicknesses, waist circumference and waist to hip ratio over the 6 month intervention period. However, there were no significant changes in high-fat food intake, moderate to vigorous activity or cardiorespiratory fitness. Support for using sedentary pursuits as a mechanism for reducing overweight in those children who are already obese is also evident in the work of Epstein et al.[73] They demonstrated more success for weight loss through reinforcing a reduction in sedentary pursuits rather than increasing physical activity. Reducing TV watching and video game usage may therefore be a useful strategy for both a population-based approach to help prevent childhood obesity and also reduce overweight in those children who are already obese.

Promoting activity in youngsters

Much more needs to be learned about how to promote more physical activity and reduce time spent in front of a TV screen for overweight and obese children. However, on current knowledge, it is clear that approaches need to be comprehensive and emphasize the development of skills necessary for behaviour change and maintain those changes. Youngsters spend almost all of their time under the influence of the home and school, so both environments need to be considered by health professionals who are working with obese children. Barlow and Dietz[63] suggested that the skills families should learn include:

- Development of awareness of current activity behaviour
- Identification of problem behaviours and obstacles to activity
- Modification of current behaviour, making a few small, permanent changes at a time and making additional changes only once the previous changes are firmly in place
- Recognition of problems that arise as the child becomes more independent or as family schedules and other changes occur

Schools can help through physical educators being sensitive to the special needs of overweight and obese children. For any particular physical task, the heavier child works harder for the same result as a lean child and it would help if this was acknowledged. Classes need to be accepting, nonthreatening and fun, and to emphasize social interaction and focus on personal improvement of skills and fitness, rather than comparison with others. It is ironic that alongside increasing obesity, we have more and more youngsters who are becoming hypersensitive about fatness. Many girls (and increasing numbers of boys), several of whom are within the optimal fat range, are using unhealthy and ineffective weight management strategies such as semi-starvation, diuretics and appetite suppressants. Teachers need to be extremely careful how they deal with issues such as overweight and place the emphasis on healthy eating and enjoyable exercise. Children who are already overweight or fat need a sensitive, individualized approach.

Table 9.4 shows several possible targets of change that have the potential to increase energy expenditure substantially.

Summary

The secular trend in overweight and obesity shows no sign of slowing down. The evidence of increasing fatness in children suggests that more adults will become obese at earlier ages over the next two or three decades, causing more human suffering and greater health care costs. This chapter has indicated that physical activity has a critical role to play in both the prevention and treatment of obesity. It is particularly pertinent in children where

Table 9.4
Packages of activity and behaviour for children.

* *Walking or cycling to school*
* *Active play at break and lunch times*
* *Sport that is attractive, regardless of ability, shape and size*
* *Active play opportunities around and outside the home*
* *Active jobs such as delivery rounds, gardening and jobbing*
* *Taking the dog for a walk every evening*
* *Active family pursuits at weekends*
* *Negotiated limits to TV viewing*
* *Using the computer/game station as a treat rather than a way of life.*

greater levels of physical activity may help prevent the development of obesity. It is also even more important for maintenance of health in those who are already overweight or obese.

Physical activity is a health behaviour similar to eating or smoking. In order to facilitate long-term behavioural change, many people need professional assistance. With regard to exercise, obese individuals often have low levels of awareness and expertise and do not have the behavioural skills necessary to maintain behavioural change. There is a clear role for the exercise specialist or health professional who has sound experience with counselling skills, educational strategies, motivational psychology and behavioural and environmental change strategies and who can apply them sensitively to this challenging and dominating health problem.

References

1   Berlin JA, Colditz GA, A meta analysis of physical activity in the prevention of coronary heart disease, *Am J Epidemiology* (1990) **132**:612–28.

2   Powell KE, Thompson PD, Casperson CJ, Kendrick JS, Physical activity and the incidence of coronary heart disease, *Ann Rev Pub Health* (1987) **8**:253–87.

3   US Department of Health and Human Services (PHS), *Physical activity and health: A Report of the Surgeon General (Executive Summary).* (Superintendent of Documents: Pittsburgh, 1996).

4   WHO, Exercise for health. WHO/FIMS Committee on Physical Activity for Health, *Bull World Health Org* (1995) **73**:135–6.

5   Killoran AJ, Fentem, P, Casperson C (eds), *Moving on: International Perspectives on Promoting Physical Activity* (Health Education Authority: London, 1994).

6   Fox KR, The influence of physical activity on mental well-being, *Public Health Nutr* (1999) **2**:411–18.

7   Blair SN, Kohl HW, Barlow CE et al, Changes in physical fitness and all-cause mortality: a prospective study of healthy and unhealthy men, *JAMA* (1995) **273**:1093–8.

8   Pratt M, Macera CA, Blanton C, Levels of physical activity and inactivity in children and adults in the United States; current evidence and research issues, *Med Sci Sport Ex* (1999) **31**:S526–33.

9   DiPietro L, Physical activity in the prevention of obesity: current evidence and research issues, *Med Sci Sport Ex* (1999) **31**:S542–6.

10   Jebb SA, Moore MS, Contribution of a sedentary lifestyle and inactivity to the etiology of overweight and obesity: current evidence and research issues, *Med Sci Sport Ex* (1999) **31**:S534–41.

11   Lee CD, Jackson AS, Blair SN, US weight guidelines: is it also important to consider cardiorespiratory fitness? *Int J Obes* (1998) **22**:S2–8.

12   Lee CD, Blair SN, Jackson AS, Cardiorespiratory fitness, body composition, and all-cause mortality in men, *Am J Clin Nutr* (1999) **69**:373–80.

13   Blair SN, Bouchard C (co-chairs), Physical activity and obesity: American College of Sports Medicine Consensus Conference, *Med Sci Sport Ex* (1999) **31**:S497.

14   National Institutes of Health and National Heart, Lung, and Blood Institute, Clinical guidelines on the identification, evaluation, and treatment of overweight and obesity in adults: the Evidence Report, *Obes Res* (1998) **6**(Suppl 2):51S–209S.

15   Rissanen A, Fogelholm M, Physical activity in the prevention and treatment of other morbid conditions and impairments associated with obesity: current evidence and research issues, *Med Sci Sport Ex* (1999) **31**:S635–45.

16   Stefanick ML, Physical activity for preventing and treating obesity-related dislipoproteinemias, *Med Sci Sport Ex* (1999) **31**:S609–18.

17   Fagard, RH, Physical activity in the prevention and treatment of hypertension in the obese, *Med Sci Sport Ex* (1999) **31**:S624–30.

18   Kelley DE, Goodpaster BH, Effects of physical activity on insulin action and glucose tolerance in obesity, *Med Sci Sport Ex* (1999) **31**:S619–23.

19   Craft LL, Landers DM, The effect of exercise on clinical depression and depression resulting from mental illness: a meta analysis, *J Sport Exerc Psycho* (1998) **20**:339–57.

20   Mutrie N, The relationship between physical activity and clinically defined depression. In: Biddle SJH, Fox KR, Boutcher SH, eds, *Physical Activity and Psychological Well-being* (Routledge: London, 2000) 46–62.

21   Fox KR, Self-esteem, self-perceptions and exercise, *Int J Sport Psychol* (2000) **31**:228–40.

22   Ballor DL, Poehlman ET, Exercise-training enhances fat-free mass preservation during diet-induced weight loss: a meta-analytical finding, *Int J Obes* (1994) **18**:35–40.

23   DiPietro L, Physical activity, body weight and adiposity: an epidemiological perspective, *Exerc Sports Sci Rev* (1995) **23**:275–304.

24   Garrow JS, Summerbell CD, Meta-analysis: effect of exercise, with or without dieting, on body composition of overweight subjects, *Eur J Clin Nutr* (1995) **49**:1–10.

25   Stefanick,ML, Exercise and weight control, *Exerc Sports Sci Rev* (1993) **21**:363–96.

26   Wilfley DE, Brownell KD, Physical activity and diet in weight loss. In: Dishman RK, ed, *Advances in Exercise Adherence* (Human Kinetics: Champaign, 1994) 361–88.

27 Wing RR, Physical activity in the treatment of the adulthood overweight and obesity: current evidence and research issues, *Med Sci Sport Ex* (1999) **31**:S547–52.

28 Ross R, Pedwell H, Rissanen J, Response of total and regional lean tissue and skeletal muscle to a program of energy restriction and resistance exercise, *Int J Obes* (1995) **19**:781–7.

29 Ross R, Janssen I, Is abdominal fat preferentially reduced in response to exercise-induced weight loss? *Med Sci Sport Ex* (1999) **31**:S568–72.

30 King AC, Tribble DL, The role of exercise in weight regulation in nonathletes, *Sports Med* (1991) **11**:331–49.

31 Pavlou KN, Krey S, Steffee WP, Exercise as an adjunct to weight loss and maintenance in moderately obese subjects, *Am J Clin Nutr* (1989) **49**:1115–23.

32 Wing RR, Epstein LH, Paternostro-Bayles et al, Exercise in a behavioural weight control programme for obese patients with type 2 (non-insulin-dependent) diabetes, *Diabetologia* (1988) **31**:902–9.

33 Svendsen OL, Hassager C, Christiansen C, Six months' follow-up on exercise added to a short-term diet in overweight postmenopausal women – effects on body composition, resting metabolic rate, cardiovascular risk factors and bone, *Int J Obes* (1994) **18**:692–8.

34 Centers for Disease Control, *Assessing Health Risks in America. The Behavioral Risk Factor Surveillance System (BRFSS) at a Glance* (Centres For Disease Control and Prevention: Atlanta, 1995).

35 Prescott-Clarke P, Primatesta P, *Health Survey for England, 1995: Findings (Vol 1)* (HMSO: London, 1997).

36 Martinez-Gonzalez MÁ, Martinez JA, Hu FB et al, Physical inactivity, sedentary lifestyle and obesity in the European Union, *Int J Obes* (1999) **23**:1192–201.

37 Schulz LO & Schoeller DA, A companion of total daily energy expenditure and body weight in healthy adults, *Am J Clin Nutr* (1994) **60**:676–81.

38 Prentice AM, Jebb S, Obesity in Britain: gluttony or sloth, *Br Med J* (1995) **311**:437–9.

39 Williamson DF, Madans J, Anda RF et al, Recreational physical activity and ten-year weight change in a US national cohort, *Int J Obes* (1993) **17**:279–86.

40 DiPietro L, Hohl HW, Barlow CE et al, Improvements in cardiorespiratory fitness attenuate age-related weight gain in healthy men and women: the Aerobics Center Longitudinal Study, *Int J Obes* (1998) **22**:55–62.

41 Ching PLYH, Willett WC, Rimm EB et al, Activity level and risk of over-weight in male health professionals, *Am J Public Health* (1996) **86**:25–30.

42 Pate RR, Pratt M, Blair SN et al, Physical activity and public health: a recommendation from the Centers for Disease Control and Prevention and the American College of Sports Medicine, *JAMA* (1995) **273**:402–8.

43 Blair SN, Hardman A, Special issue: physical activity, health and well-being – an international consensus conference, *Res Quart Exerc Sport* (1995) **66**:4.

44 Haskell WL, Dose–response issues from a biological perspective. In: Bouchard C, Shephard RJ, Stephens T, eds, *Physical Activity, Fitness and Health: International Proceedings and Consensus Statement* (Human Kinetics: Champaign, 1994) 1030–9.

45 Haskell WL, Health consequences of physical activity: understanding and challenges regarding

dose–response, *Med Sci Sports Exerc* (1994b) **26**:649–60.

46 Jakicic JM, Wing RR, Butler BA, Robertson RJ, Prescribing exercise in multiple short bouts versus one continuous bout, *Int J Obes* (1995) **19**:893–901.

47 Jakicic JM, Winters C, Lang W, Wing RR, Effects of intermittent exercise and use of home exercise equipment on adherence, weight loss, and fitness in overweight women: a randomized trial, *JAMA* (1999) **282**:1554–60.

48 Blundell JE, King NA, Effects of exercise on appetite control: loose coupling between energy expenditure and energy intake, *Int J Obes* (1998) **22**(Suppl 2):S22–8.

49 Blundell JE, King NA, Physical activity and regulation of food intake: current evidence, *Med Sci Sport Ex* (1999) **31**:S573–83.

50 Gwinup G, Effect of exercise alone on the weight of obese women, *Arch Intern Med* (1975) **135**:676–80.

51 Hill JO, Schlundt DG, Sbroccot T et al, Evaluation of an alternating-calorie diet with and without exercise in the treatment of obesity, *Am J Clin Nutr* (1989) **50**:248–54.

52 Biddle SJH, Fox KR, Motivation for physical activity and weight management, *Int J Obes* (1998) **22**:S39–47.

53 Marcus B, Simkin L, Rossi J, Pinto B, Longitudinal shifts in employees' stages and process of exercise behaviour change. *Am J Health Promotion* (1996) **10**:195–201.

54 Fox KR, A clinical approach to exercise in the morbidly obese. In: Wadden T, Van Itallie T, eds, *Treatment of the Seriously Obese Patient* (Guilford Press: New York, 1992) 354–82.

55 Rollnick S, Behaviour change in practice: targeting individuals, *Int J Obes* (1996) **20**:S22–6.

56 Fahlberg LL, Fahlberg LA, From treatment to health enhancement: psychosocial considerations in the exercise components of health promotion programs, *Sport Psychol* (1990) **4**:168–79.

57 Gillet PA, Self-reported factors influencing exercise adherence in overweight women, *Nursing Res* (1988) **37**:25–9.

58 Anderson JP, Fox KR, A social support scale for exercise in a clinical setting: preliminary evidence of construct validity, *J Sports Sci* (1998) **16**:71.

59 Perri MG, McAdoo WG, McAllister DA et al, Enhancing the efficacy of behavior therapy for obesity: effects of aerobic exercise and a multicomponent treatment maintenance program, *J Consult Clin Psychol* (1986) **54**:670–5.

60 Flegal KM, The obesity epidemic in children and adults: current evidence and research issues, *Med Sci Sports Exerc* (1999) **31**:S509–14.

61 Reilly JJ, Dorosty AH, Epidemic of obesity in UK children, *Lancet* (1999) **354**:1874–5.

62 Prentice AM, Body mass index standards for children, *Br Med J* (1998) **317**:1401–2.

63 Barlow SM, Dietz WH, Obesity evaluation and treatment: expert committee recommendations, *Pediatrics* (1998) **102**:e29.

64 Sallis JF, Patrick K, Physical activity guidelines for adolescents: consensus statement, *Pediatr Exerc Sci* (1994) **6**:302–14.

65 Biddle SJH, Sallis JF, Cavill NA, *Young and active? Young People and Health Enhancing Physical Activity: Evidence and Implications* (Health Education Authority: London, 1998).

66 Epstein LH, Goldfield GS, Physical activity in the treatment of childhood overweight and obesity: current evidence and research issues, *Med Sci Sports Exerc* (1999) **31**:S553–S559.

67 Epstein LH, Wing RR, Koeske R et al, A comparison of lifestyle change and programmed aerobic exercise on weight and fitness changes in obese children, *Behav Ther* (1982) **13**:651–65.

68 Epstein LH, Valoski AM, Wing RR et al, Ten-year outcomes of behavioural family-based treatment for childhood obesity, *Health Psychol* (1994) **13**:373–83.

69 Epstein LH, Wing RR, Koeske et al, A comparison of lifestyle exercise, aerobic exercise and calisthenics on weight loss in obese children, *Behav Ther* (1985) **16**:345–56.

70 Dietz WH, Strasburger VC, Children, adolescents and television, *Curr Prob Pediatr* (1991) **21**:8–31.

71 Gortmaker SL, Must A, Sobol AM et al, Television viewing as a cause of increasing obesity amont children in the United States 1986–1990, *Arch Pediatr Adolesc Med* (1996) **150**:356–62.

72 Robinson TN, Reducing children's television viewing to prevent obesity: a randomized controlled trial, *JAMA* (1999) **282**:1561–7.

73 Epstein LH, Valoski AM, Vara LS et al, Effects of decreasing sedentary behavior and increasing activity on weight change in obese children, *Health Psychol* (1995) **14**:109–15.

Pharmacological approaches

John Wilding

10

Introduction

Drug treatment of obesity has had a chequered, and at times controversial history, and it is important to consider the currently available treatments in the light of this previous experience. Many of the older agents were never rigorously evaluated in the way that would be considered the minimum standard today, and the evidence of their effectiveness was often based on small, short-term studies, with little attempt to investigate effects on the co-morbidities of obesity. Some of these agents also turned out to have serious adverse effects, which has resulted in their withdrawal for safety reasons. Two new drugs (orlistat and sibutramine) have recently been approved for use in many countries and, at present, seem to be at least as effective, and safer, than the older drugs; furthermore, there are many more data about their effectiveness in terms of the co-morbidities of obesity. Nevertheless, as clinicians it is important to ensure that such drugs are used in an appropriate and responsible manner, using the best available evidence. This chapter will briefly describe the range of possible options in the pharmacotherapy of obesity, discuss when it might be appropriate to consider drug treatment, assess the effects on body weight and co-morbidities and, finally, look towards the future to see what might be available in another few years.

Possible pharmacological approaches to weight loss

At the most simplistic level, a drug can cause weight loss only by reducing energy intake or by increasing energy expenditure. In practice, there are several ways of achieving these goals, and some agents have effects on both sides of the energy balance equation. Energy intake can be reduced either by influencing the mechanisms in the central nervous system that control appetite, by making a subject feel less hungry, or more satiated after a meal; the majority of older appetite suppressants and the newer agent sibutramine work in this way.[1] An alternative approach is to reduce absorption of nutrients – the latter will only be effective, however, if there is no compensatory increase in food consumption. Orlistat, which decreases fat absorption, is the only effective agent in this class.[2] Modifying carbohydrate absorption, for example with an α-glucosidase inhibitor such as acarbose, does not influence body weight.[3] Energy expenditure can also be regulated in a number of ways: centrally, most probably mediated by an increase in activity of the sympathetic nervous system, that in turn increases metabolic rate in target tissues, or directly

through an effect on the target tissue to increase energy use (Figure 10.1). Drugs have been developed that work at each of these levels, although not all have yet reached clinical practice, and many have so far only been evaluated in animal models.[4,5] Because the regulatory systems that control food intake and energy expenditure are closely linked both anatomically and functionally, many of the drugs that work in the central nervous system are able to influence both sides of the energy balance equation. For example, it has been found that sibutramine, and to some extent the older, centrally-acting drugs such as the fenfluramines, have effects on satiety and energy expenditure, although the relative importance of these effects in terms of efficacy is not yet known.[6]

When is drug treatment for obesity useful?

Not all obese patients want, or will benefit from drug treatment, and it is important to target those who are most likely to benefit, avoid using drugs where it is not appropriate, and also to recognize when treatment is not working, and discontinue the drug if this is the case. At present it is most appropriate to consider drug treatment in patients who are well motivated, but have not been able to achieve a target weight loss of 10% despite supervised efforts to modify their lifestyle through diet, exercise and behavioural

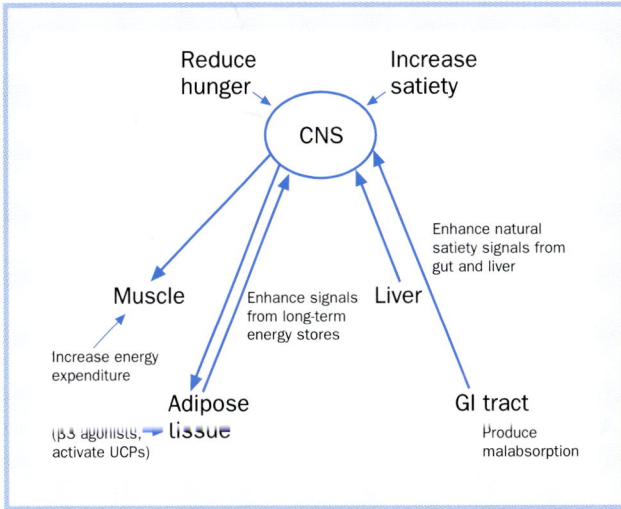

Figure 10.1
Potential targets for obesity pharmacotherapy.

change.[7] Many authorities advocate targeting patients with co-morbidities such as diabetes, hypertension and dyslipidaemia; whilst these patients will certainly stand to benefit from weight loss, this is not a good reason to deny others intervention, as many obese patients will have significant symptoms as a result of obesity, and may well benefit in a whole range of other ways, such as improvement in cancer and diabetes risk, and improvement in non-specific symptoms. Drug therapy should be avoided in patients who have evidence of an eating disorder such as bulimia. It is good practice to avoid offering drug therapy to patients who are seeking a quick fix for their obesity, without giving them an opportunity to try and lose weight through a structured programme of diet and exercise first; such patients are likely to be disappointed. Finally, drugs should not be given to patients who are not obese or in those with known contraindications to the drug being considered.

How should pharmacotherapy be used?

Weight loss or weight maintenance?

Conventional wisdom suggests that obese patients will usually be considered for drug treatment as an aid to weight loss; however, whilst many patients are able to lose modest amounts of weight in the short term through changes to diet and physical activity, the greatest challenge is in fact maintaining weight loss long term. There is now some evidence from clinical trials from the newer obesity drug treatments, that they may be useful in helping to maintain weight loss achieved through other means as well as inducing weight loss. Whether or not weight loss or weight maintenance is considered the primary goal of therapy, it is clear from trials of every agent studied so far that the emphasis needs to shift from weight loss to weight maintenance after about 6 months of treatment, as no drug is likely to produce continued weight loss after this period of time. The reasons for this are complex, but may be related to the fall in energy requirements that occurs with weight loss, resulting in the individual reaching a new 'set-point' for body weight after a certain period of time. For this reason it is important to consider carefully the criteria that should be used to judge the efficacy of any pharmacological treatment for obesity.

Criteria for success

Given the chronic nature of obesity, the tendency for body weight to rise steadily throughout adult life, and the presence of co-morbidities that are improved by a modest weight loss of 5–10%, several groups have considered the criteria for successful obesity pharmacotherapy.[7,8] At present the arguments

are based around expectations of improvements in morbidity and mortality from a variety of obesity-related conditions, mainly derived from epidemiological data and observed changes in surrogate end-points such as lipids, blood pressure and diabetes status with drug treatment. Ultimately it is hoped that firm evidence of long-term benefit would be used as a criterion, but this information is not yet available for any therapy. Based on this information, the Royal College of Physicians in the UK and SIGN in Scotland have suggested that a weight loss of 5% after 3 months' therapy indicates that the treatment is successful; drug therapy should be discontinued in patients who do not achieve this degree of weight loss. It is also stated that weight gain on therapy (an amount is not specified) indicates that treatment is failing and again suggests that treatment should be stopped. This latter statement needs careful consideration in individual patients, as it clearly depends how much weight has been regained, in proportion to the initial weight loss achieved (Figure 10.2).

Duration of treatment

At present there are few clinical trial data on the use of any obesity pharmacotherapy for longer than 2 years, so the licence for newer drugs, such as sibutramine and orlistat, is limited to 2 years in many countries. Whilst this is probably a sensible approach given the

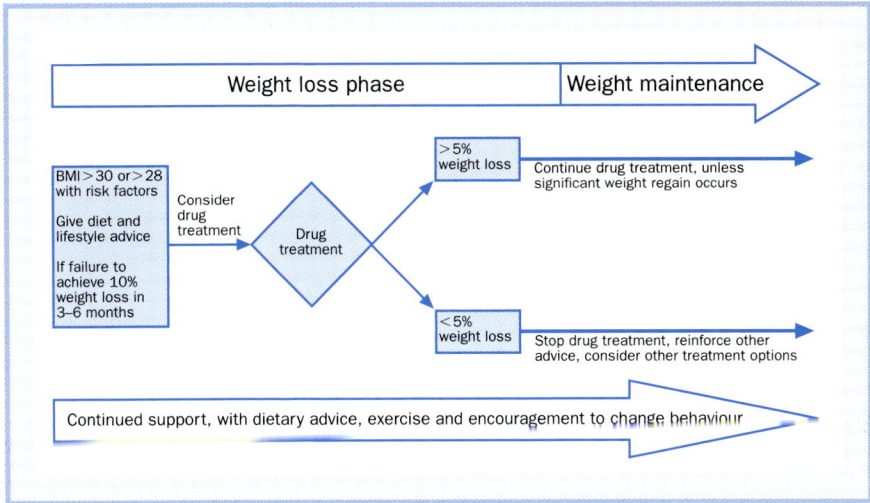

Figure 10.2
When should obesity pharmacotherapy be used, and when should it be stopped? (Adapted from RCP guidelines 1998.[7])

lack of data on the safety and efficacy of these drugs beyond 2 years of therapy, there is a strong case for considering whether obesity drugs could perhaps be used long term, at least in some patients. Firstly, it is well recognized that once drug treatment is stopped, then weight regain usually occurs. This is perhaps unsurprising, and is analogous to the situation in many other chronic conditions such as diabetes, hypertension and hyperlipidaemia that require lifelong therapy. Nevertheless, some patients will succeed in maintaining a lower weight without treatment, and a pragmatic approach, given

the current limitations on duration of drug treatment, is to withdraw therapy once the licensed treatment period is over, and continue to give dietary and exercise advice. If weight regain begins to occur, then re-introduction of treatment can be considered, provided it is within the licence of the drug.

Obesity pharmacotherapy

This section will describe the pharmacology, efficacy and effects on obesity-related illness of a range of drug treatments for obesity, including those that are now withdrawn from use, and commonly used licensed and unlicensed medication. Finally, agents that might become available in the near future will be briefly discussed.

Older and withdrawn drugs

Although some of the drugs described in this section are no longer available, many obese patients will have previously used these agents, so it is important for physicians treating obesity to be aware of their pharmacology, particularly with regard to the possibility of late recognition of adverse events.

Phentermine

Phentermine is a centrally-acting drug that is a sympathomimetic. It is thought to suppress appetite, and possibly have a modest thermogenic effect. It has been evaluated in trials of up to 36 weeks' duration as monotherapy and is effective at producing weight loss of up to 12.2 kg (vs 4.8 kg on placebo).[9] There are few data on effects on obesity co-morbidities. Phentermine may induce dependency, and has significant CNS side effects such as irritability and anxiety, consistent with its central sympathomimetic mode of action. It remains available in the USA, but its licence in the European Union was withdrawn in May 2001.

Fenfluramine and dexfenfluramine

These two drugs (dexfenfluramine is the active D-isomer of fenfluramine, which is a racemic mixture) enhance serotonin release from neurons and other tissues. Although effective at producing weight loss, principally by acting on the hypothalamus to reduce appetite,[10] they have now been withdrawn because they were found to produce carcinoid-like valvular heart lesions in many patients, resulting in mitral and aortic regurgitation, which in some cases required valve replacement.[11] This side effect was particularly common in patients who were also taking phentermine, although valve defects have not been associated with phentermine monotherapy. The fenfluramines have also been associated with primary pulmonary hypertension; although the incidence of this side effect is low (18 per million; compared to 6 per million for the population), it may only become apparent some years after taking the drug.[12] It is a relentlessly progressive condition, and can result in severe cardiac and respiratory failure that can only be effectively treated by heart–lung transplantation.

Diethylpropion

There are few data on this centrally-acting agent, which has only been tested in short-term trials. Although it is more effective than placebo at producing weight loss, there have been some concerns because of its stimulatory effect on the central nervous system.

Drugs not licensed for obesity treatment

Ephedrine and caffeine

A number of small studies have been published using a combination of ephedrine and caffeine, used for up to 1 year for weight loss and weight maintenance. Ephedrine is a centrally acting sympathomimetic with anorectic and thermogenic activity. Its effects are potentiated by caffeine. Side effects include a rise in heart rate and blood pressure and a transient rise in glucose. Although this combination does produce greater weight loss than placebo, and may have a protein-sparing effect, the overall weight loss over placebo is modest (less than 2 kg in most studies) and neither drug alone, nor the combination, is licensed for the treatment of obesity.

Fluoxetine

Fluoxetine is a serotonin reuptake inhibitor that is licensed as an antidepressant; it was observed to cause weight loss in a number of clinical trials, and has been evaluated in several studies in uncomplicated obesity, and in obese patients with type 2 diabetes.[13] Most of these studies have shown it to be effective at producing some initial weight loss,[14] but this

is not maintained long term, as most patients regain the lost weight within 6 to 12 months, despite continuing treatment. Hence fluoxetine is not licensed or recommended for the treatment of obesity.

Currently available obesity drugs

The two newest agents available for obesity treatment, sibutramine and orlistat, have been much more extensively evaluated than any of the treatments described above, in terms of duration of treatment, and for their effects on obesity-related co-morbidities. However, it should be noted that neither drug has been formally evaluated for use for longer than 2 years, nor are there long-term outcome data on the effectiveness of these treatments.

Orlistat

Orlistat is a pancreatic intestinal lipase inhibitor that reduces the absorption of dietary fat in a dose-dependent manner. At the therapeutic dose of 120 mg three times daily, it blocks the absorption of about 30% of dietary triglyceride, resulting in an energy loss of about 200 kcal per day for an individual on an average diet of 2200 kcal per day with 40% of the calories from fat.[15]

Side effects

The undigested fat is lost in the stool, which may produce steatorrhoea; patients may complain of loose stools, anal leakage or, occasionally, faecal incontinence. Fortunately, in clinical trials such adverse events became less common with longer duration of treatment.[16] This has been attributed to patients learning to avoid meals that are high in fat; given that low-fat diets may themselves help weight loss, this may well contribute to the therapeutic effects of orlistat treatment. The only other adverse effects reported in clinical trials are modest reductions in circulating concentrations of fat-soluble vitamins (A, D, E and K), and beta-carotene. However, concentrations only rarely fell below the normal range, and no patients developed clinical vitamin deficiency. Other indices of vitamin status such as INR, PTH and bone density were not affected. Orlistat is not appreciably absorbed systemically (<1%).

Contraindications and interactions
Orlistat should not be used in patients with malabsorption, cholestasis or known hypersensitivity to the drug. It should be avoided during breastfeeding and is not licensed for use in children. It has been tested for interactions with a wide range of commonly used medication, and no significant drug interactions or effects on absorption have been found.

Efficacy: weight loss
Several randomized, double-blind, placebo-controlled trials of orlistat for weight loss of up to 2 years' duration have been conducted, and published in full. Similar protocols have been used for each of these studies, comprising a 4-week run-in period, a 12-month treatment period on active treatment or placebo, combined with advice to follow a 500–800 kcal deficit diet (the exact deficit being calculated from estimated energy expenditure, using standard equations) and a second 12-month period with relaxation of the diet with the aim of encouraging weight maintenance, rather than continued weight loss. In both studies, some patients were crossed over from orlistat to placebo, or from placebo to orlistat for the second year.

In the European study,[17] patients had an average BMI of 36 kg/m^2 and three-quarters were female. The mean weight loss at 1 year was 10.2%, compared to 6.1% in the placebo group. During the second year, some weight regain occurred in both groups, but this was less in those patients treated with orlistat (Figure 10.3a). Patients who crossed over from placebo to orlistat lost additional weight and those switched from orlistat to placebo regained most, but not all of the additional weight lost. Overall, of patients completing 2 years of orlistat treatment, 57.1% maintained a weight loss of at least 5%, compared with 37.4% of placebo-treated patients.

Very similar results were reported in a 2-year study carried out in the United States;[18] some patients in this study received orlistat, 60 mg tds, but this was less efficacious, and is

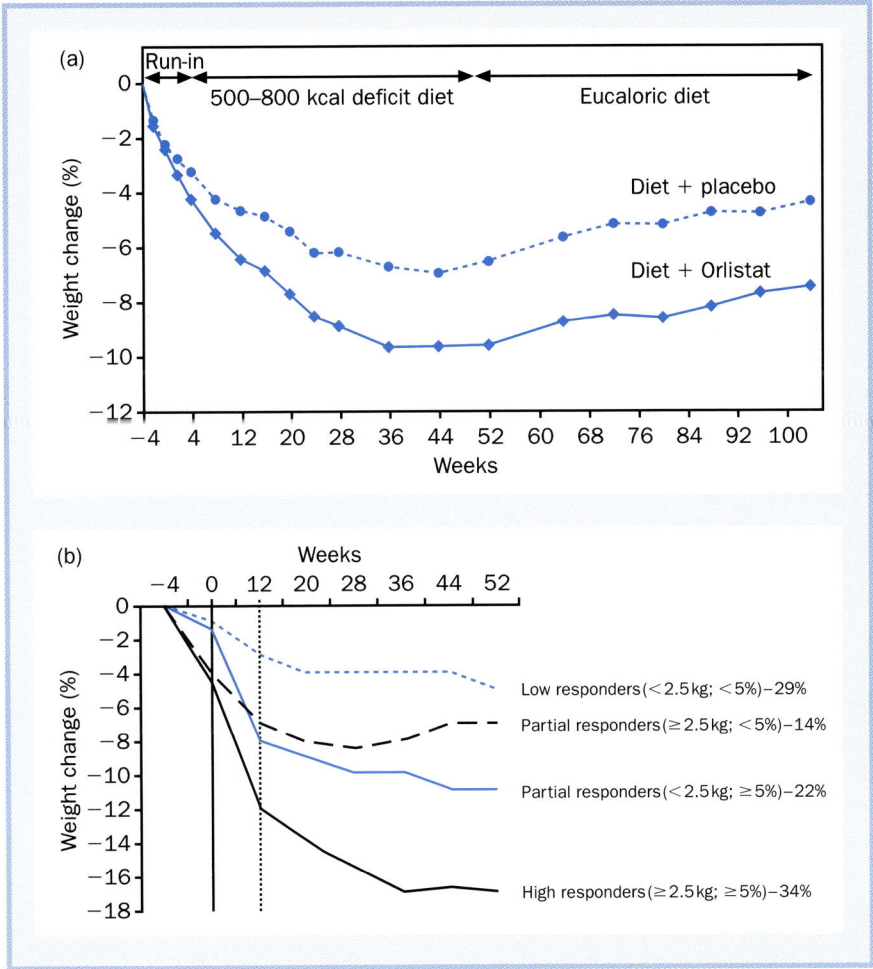

Figure 10.3
Orlistat: (a) average weight loss and weight regain during weight maintenance. (b) Final weight loss achieved as categorized by weight loss during the run-in period showing 'responders' who would be eligible for treatment under the European licence, having lost 2.5 kg during run-in, and who achieved a 5% weight loss during the first 3 months of treatment.[19]

less than the currently recommended dose of 120 mg tds, so these results will not be discussed further. These studies were conducted in centres specializing in obesity management, but one study has been reported where the trial was carried out in primary care centres in the USA.[20] In this study, the patient population was similar, but the intervention consisted of videos on behavioural change and leaflets given every 3 months; no dietitians or behavioural counsellors were used in this study. Weight loss was slightly less than seen in the secondary care centres (7.94 kg vs 4.14 kg), and 34% vs 24% maintained a weight loss of at least 5% over 2 years. Nevertheless, this study does indicate that orlistat treatment can be effective when given with fairly basic advice about diet and behavioural change.

One further analysis relevant to weight loss has been reported. This looked at whether subsequent weight loss can be predicted, either from the weight loss that occurred during the run-in period, or during the first 3 months of therapy. Patients who lost at least 2.5 kg during the 4-week run-in period, and who subsequently lost 5% of body weight in the first 3 months of treatment, achieved an average weight loss at 12 months of over 17%. These patients (34% of those in the trials) would be the only subjects eligible to receive long-term orlistat treatment under the current European licensing conditions for the drug (Figure 10.3b). Not surprisingly, those who achieved neither criterion did relatively poorly in terms of weight loss, and those who achieved one of the two criteria had an intermediate degree of success. These observations highlight the point that for orlistat to be maximally effective, patients need to be well motivated to lose weight, which can be demonstrated by showing the ability to lose some weight prior to starting drug treatment, and that if the patient is not losing significant amounts of weight on treatment, then an alternative approach should be considered.

Efficacy: co-morbidities

In each of the studies described above, effects of orlistat treatment on cardiovascular risk factors such as lipids, blood pressure and insulin resistance have been reported. A number of studies aimed at treating subjects with at least one cardiovascular risk factor have been reported, and one study in diabetic patients has been published in full.[21]

The reduction in lipids seen with orlistat in patients without overt dyslipidaemia (a 0.12 mmol fall in cholesterol at the end of year 2 and a 12.7% fall in the LDL/HDL ratio), is modest, but is greater than might be expected for the degree of weight loss; this could be due either to a specific effect to reduce cholesterol absorption, or to the reinforcement of a low-fat diet. Blood pressure falls were modest in patients without hypertension (around 1–2 mm Hg difference

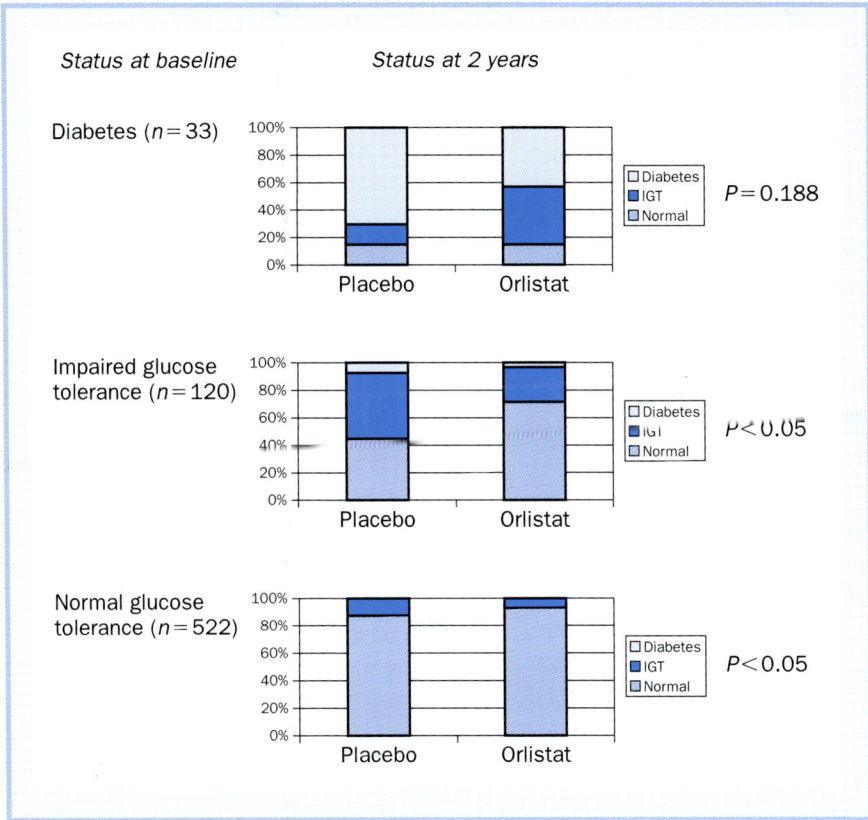

Figure 10.4
Effect of 2 years of orlistat treatment on glucose tolerance. (Data from Heymsfield et al 2000.[24])

from placebo). Fasting insulin and insulin resistance also improve,[22] and a recent report based on a meta-analysis of some of the trial data suggests that patients with impaired glucose tolerance are more likely to improve to normal and less likely to deteriorate during

a 2-year follow up. Similarly patients with normal glucose tolerance are less likely to develop impaired glucose tolerance[23] (Figure 10.4).

There are few available data on the effects of orlistat on other obesity-related co-morbidities, such as sleep apnoea, osteoarthritis, dyspnoea and quality of life.

In summary, orlistat can help promote weight loss when used in combination with moderate calorie restriction. It is most effective in well-motivated patients who have shown they are able to lose some weight through diet and lifestyle modification. The additional weight loss seen with orlistat therapy has beneficial effects on cardiovascular risk factors and diabetes risk, but the long-term cost-effectiveness of this approach to risk factor management remains unproven.

Sibutramine

Sibutramine is a noradrenaline and serotonin reuptake inhibitor; together with its active metabolites (M1 and M2) it increases the availability of these two neurotransmitters at sites in the hypothalamus that are involved in the regulation of food intake and energy expenditure. It has been evaluated at doses of up to 30 mg daily, although the usual therapeutic dose is 5–15 mg taken once daily. Sibutramine is thought to reduce body weight by both reducing food intake (particularly by enhancing satiety) and by increasing energy expenditure by activating the sympathetic nervous system.[23,25]

Side effects

Side effects of sibutramine that were reported more commonly than placebo in clinical trials included dry mouth, insomnia, anxiety and constipation. In clinical trials these side effects only rarely (<1%), led to withdrawal from the study. There is also a modest increase in heart rate of 4 to 6 beats per minute with sibutramine, and some patients will have a rise in blood pressure (mean 2–3 mm Hg), although this is partially offset by the fall in blood pressure that occurs with weight loss.[26]

Sibutramine is pharmacologically distinct from previously available drugs, such as the fenfluramines, which are serotonin-releasing agents, and there is no evidence that its use results in cardiac valvular abnormalities or primary pulmonary hypertension. Studies have also shown that it does not have addictive or euphoric properties, and is unlikely to be used as a drug of abuse.

Contraindications and interactions

Because of the concerns regarding effects on heart rate and blood pressure, sibutramine is contraindicated in patients with a history of cardiac failure, arrhythmias or ischaemic heart disease. It should also not be given to patients with uncontrolled hypertension. Other contraindications are concomitant or recent use of monoamine oxidase inhibitors, other centrally acting anorectic drugs or sympathomimetic agents (including common 'cold cures' such as pseudoephedrine), severe hepatic or renal dysfunction and patients with a history of seizures. Sibutramine is metabolized by cytochrome P450(3A4) and may interact with other drugs metabolized by this pathway, including cimetidine, erythromycin and ketoconazole.

Efficacy: weight loss

Several short-term (mainly dose-ranging studies) and long-term (1–2 year) studies with sibutramine have been conducted and reported in the literature. These have all used a range of additional strategies to assist with weight loss, including basic dietary advice, individually tailored advice based on calculated metabolic rate, the use of very-low-calorie diets and exercise advice. Sibutramine was effective at producing weight loss in doses above 5 mg daily in a 24-week dose-ranging study. In this study, weight loss was proportional to dose; patients receiving 10 and 15 mg of sibutramine (doses that are used in clinical practice) achieved weight losses of 6.1 and 7.4%, respectively, compared to a placebo weight loss of 1.2%.[27] In a 12-month trial conducted in UK general practice, the mean weight loss was 5% at a 10 mg dose and 8% at 15 mg. Proportionally more patients achieved a weight loss of at least 5% and 10% in the active treatment group. When used as a treatment to enhance weight maintenance after weight loss following a very-low-calorie diet, sibutramine (10 mg) treatment resulted in an additional weight loss of 5.2 kg compared to a 0.5 kg gain in the placebo group. When the 4-week VLCD-induced weight loss of 7.7 kg before the study was also

considered, 86% of patients achieved a 5% weight loss at the end of 12 months' treatment[26] (Figure 10.5).

The STORM (Sibutramine Trial in Obesity Reduction and Maintenance) study was recently reported.[28] This was a 2-year study, conducted in uncomplicated obese patients and employed a unique study design whereby all patients received sibutramine 10 mg daily for 6 months. Following this, patients who had lost at least 5% of weight from baseline were randomized to sibutramine (10, 15 or 20 mg, titrated according to weight loss) or placebo, with the aim of maintaining weight lost. All patients received intensive advice on diet (every 2 weeks) and physical activity. The average maintained weight loss at 2 years (LOCF analysis) was 8.9 kg in the sibutramine group, and 4.9 kg in the placebo group. This was associated with significant improvements in lipids and insulin resistance and, as expected, small increases in heart rate and blood pressure.

Efficacy: co-morbidities

Within the above trials the effects of sibutramine treatment on cardiovascular risk factors, such as lipids and blood pressure, have also been assessed, together with a separate series of studies in diabetic patients. For example, in the VLCD study there was a lowering of LDL cholesterol, an increase in HDL cholesterol resulting in a −0.6 improvement in the total cholesterol/HDL cholesterol ratio in the active treatment group,

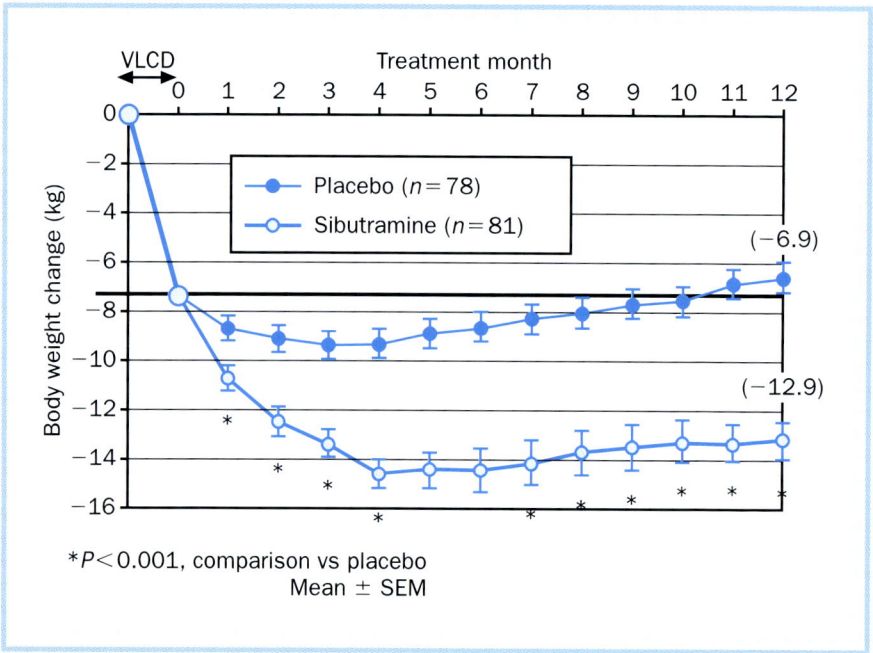

Figure 10.5
Use of pharmacotherapy for weight maintenance – sibutramine following a VLCD. (Adapted from Apfelbaum et al.[27])

compared to a -0.1 change in the placebo group. Blood pressure rose slightly (by 1.5 mm Hg) in the sibutramine group, and fell slightly (by 1.9 mm Hg) in the active treatment group. A study in hypertensive patients suggested that the drug is safe to use on obese patients with hypertension, although about 5.4% of patients had to be withdrawn because of poor control of blood pressure, compared with 1.3% of placebo-treated patients.[29] A 3-month study in diabetic patients treated with diet and a variety of oral hypoglycaemic agents showed significantly greater weight loss, and a 0.3% fall in glycated haemoglobin compared to placebo.[30] Studies in diabetic patients treated with diet, sulphonylureas and metformin and in hyperlipidaemic patients have been conducted, but the results have not yet been reported in full.[31] As with orlistat, there are few published data on the effects on other obesity-related co-morbidities, but the effects on lipids and improvements in control of diabetes are encouraging.

Combination therapy

Given the availability of two drugs with different modes of action, it is inevitable that they will be tried in combination, as is commonly the case with drugs for hypertension and diabetes. One small placebo-controlled study suggested that there was no additional benefit to adding orlistat after 1 year of sibutramine treatment,[32] but a formal study combining the two treatments has not been carried out. At present this combination is contraindicated in the license of both drugs, and *is not* recommended by any of the published guidelines on obesity treatment Perhaps of more clinical relevance will be a carefully controlled study of the sequential use of sibutramine and orlistat.

The future

Although the newer drugs described above are a real advance, and are able to achieve clinically worthwhile weight loss in a significant number of patients, it is clear they are not a panacea for the problems of obesity. Many patients, particularly those with more severe obesity, will still be at significant risk of obesity-related complications even if treatment achieves the current modest criteria that are deemed to indicate success, and the side effects may deter some patients from treatment. Hence there is a need for new agents that are able to help weight loss in a safe and effective way. In recent years there have been many advances in the

understanding of how weight and energy balance are regulated, and these are beginning to bear fruit, in terms of new drugs that are being tested in animal models and in humans.[33] Some of these are briefly described below.

Leptin

Leptin is an adipocyte-derived hormone that is produced in proportion to body fat content. It acts on receptors in the hypothalamus to reduce food intake. Absence of leptin or the presence of a defective leptin receptor results in a syndrome of severe obesity in animal models and in humans. Hence leptin seems an attractive means to treat obesity. One clinical trial with recombinant human leptin has been reported. The results are disappointing, with only minimal weight loss seen at 3 months.[34] Subjects with lower baseline leptin appeared to respond slightly better; nevertheless, the results fall well short of the weight loss seen with existing agents. Although more potent analogues may be more effective, the current understanding of leptin physiology suggests that whilst absence, or very low concentrations, of this hormone indicate that it is important physiologically, the dose–response curve is flat once concentrations reach the levels typically seen in healthy lean individuals; obese individuals already have high leptin concentrations and raising these further does not seem to produce an additional biological effect on appetite or body weight.

New centrally-acting drugs

There are now over 50 known neurotransmitters and other endogenous brain chemicals that can influence appetite and/or energy expenditure. The majority are inhibitory and may therefore be having a nonspecific effect, whereas others increase appetite. In general, those that decrease appetite tend to increase thermogenesis and vice versa. Most of these have been considered as possible pharmacological agents for obesity treatment, but particular attention has focused on stimulatory neurotransmitters, such as neuropeptide Y (looking for antagonists) and those transmitters that are targets of leptin action, such as the melanocortin-4 receptor.[35] A number of agents that are dopamine agonists have demonstrated weight loss in early clinical trials. Agonists at the cholecystokinin receptor, that mainly act to increase satiety, have shown promise in preclinical studies, and early clinical studies in humans suggest they reduced food intake during test meals, although long-term data are currently lacking.

Drugs that increase energy expenditure

The most studied group of drugs in this group is the β3-adrenoceptor agonists.[36] Activation of the β3 adrenoceptor in obese rodents turns on an uncoupling protein in brown adipose tissue, resulting in increased heat production. These drugs are effective at producing weight loss in animal models, but agents developed to date have significant cross-reactivity with other adrenoceptors in humans, resulting in side effects such as tachycardia and tremor; new agents are being developed that are selective for human β3 receptors, and the clinical trials of these are awaited. Another approach, which would have the same effect, would be to activate the uncoupling proteins directly. This idea is theoretically attractive, but no suitable drugs have yet been developed.

Conclusions

Better understanding of the control of energy balance, a reappraisal of achievable treatment goals and stricter criteria for evaluation are leading to a change in attitudes towards the use of pharmacotherapy in obesity. The drugs now available have had to pass strict tests of efficacy and safety before being used in humans; similar criteria are likely to be applied to any new therapy. Obesity therapy has increased in respectability, but before it is widely accepted into mainstream clinical practice, it is likely that further evidence of long-term benefit and cost-effectiveness will be required. Nevertheless, patients who do achieve clinically significant weight loss demonstrate improvement in symptoms, cardiovascular risk factors and quality of life. It would therefore seem reasonable to offer such treatment to such patients who are able to benefit.

References

1 Hansen DL, Toubro S, Stock MJ, Macdonald IA, Astrup A, The effect of sibutramine on energy expenditure and appetite during chronic treatment without dietary restriction, *Int J Obesity* (1999) **23:**1016–24.

2 Drent ML, van derVeen EA, Lipase inhibition – a novel concept in the treatment of obesity, *Int J Obesity* (1993) **17:**241–4.

3 Holman RR, Cull CA, Turner RC, A randomized double-blind trial of acarbose in type 2 diabetes shows improved glycemic control over 3 years (UK Prospective Diabetes Study 44), *Diabetes Care* (1999) **22:**960–4.

4 Wilding JPH, Widdowson PS, Williams G, Neurobiology, *Br Med Bull* (1997) **53:**286–306.

5 Finer N, Present and future pharmacological approaches, *Br Med Bull* (1997) **53:**409–32.

6 Hansen DL, Toubro S, Stock MJ, Macdonald IA, Astrup A, Thermogenic effects of sibutramine in humans, *Am J Clin Nutr* (1998) **68:**1180–6.

7 Royal College of Physicians. Clinical management of overweight and obese patients, with particular reference to the use of drugs, 1998.

8 Obesity in Scotland: Integrating Prevention with Weight Management, 8, 1996. Edinburgh, SIGN.

9 Munro JF, MacCuish AC, Wilson EM, Duncan LJP, Comparison of continuous and intermittent anorectic therapy in obesity, *Br Med J* (1968) **1:**352–4.

10 Wilding JPH, Gilbey SG, Jones PM, Mannan MM, Ghatei MA, Bloom SR, Dexfenfluramine treatment and hypothalamic neuropeptides in diet-induced obesity in rats, *Peptides* (1992) **13:**557–63.

11 Connolly HM, Crary JL, McGoon MD et al, Valvular heart disease associated with fenfluramine–phentermine, *N Engl J Med* (1997) **337:**581–8.

12 Abenhaim I, Moride Y, Brenot F, Appetite suppressant drugs and the risk of primary pulmonary hypertension, *N Engl J Med* (1996) **335:**609–16.

13 Connolly VM, Gallagher A, Kesson CM, A study of fluoxetine in obese elderly patients with type 2 diabetes, *Diabet Med* (1995) **12:**416–8.

14 Goldstein DJ, Rampey AH, Enas GG, Potvin JH, Fludzinski LLA, Levine LR, Fluoxetine – a randomized clinical-trial in the treatment of obesity, *Int J Obesity* (1994) **18:**129–35.

15 Hartmann D, Hussain Y, Guzelhan C, Odink J, Effect on dietary-fat absorption of orlistat, administered at different times relative to meal intake, *Br J Clin Pharmacol* (1993) **36:**266–70.

16 Sjostrom L, Rissanen A, Andersen T et al, Randomised placebo-controlled trial of orlistat for weight loss and prevention of weight regain in obese patients, *Lancet* (1998) **352:**167–72.

17 Sjostrom L, Rissanen A, Andersen T et al, Weight loss and prevention of weight regain in obese patients: a 2-year, European, randomised trial of orlistat, *Lancet* (1998) **352:**167–72.

18 Davidson MH, Hauptman J, DiGirolamo M et al, Weight control and risk factor reduction in obese subjects treated for 2 years with orlistat – a randomized controlled trial, *JAMA* (1999) **281:**235–42.

19 Rissanen A, Sjostrom L, Rossner S, Early weight

loss with orlistat as a predictor of long-term success in obesity treatment, *Int J Obesity* (1999) Suppl, S174, Abstract 577.

20 Hauptman J, Lucas C, Boldrin MN, Collins H, Segal KR, Orlistat in the long-term treatment of obesity in primary care settings, *Arch Fam Med* (2000) 9:160–7.

21 Hollander PA, Elbein SC, Hirsch IB et al, Role of orlistat in the treatment of obese patients with type 2 diabetes – a 1-year randomized double-blind study, *Diabetes Care* (1998) 21:1288–94.

22 Wilding JPH, Orlistat-induced weight loss improves insulin resistance in obese patients, *Diabetologia* (1999) 42(Suppl 1):807.

23 Heymsfield SB, Segal KR, Hauptmann J et al, Effects of weight loss with orlistat on glucose tolerance and progression to impaired glucose tolerance and type 2 diabetes in obese adults, *Arch Intern Med* (2000) 160:1321–6.

24 Halford JCG, Heal DJ, Blundell JE, Investigation of a new potential antiobesity drug, sibutramine, using the behavioral satiety sequence, *Appetite* (1994) 23:306–7.

25 Connoley IP, Frost I, Heal DJ, Stock MJ, Role of beta-adrenoceptors in mediating the thermogenic effects of sibutramine, *Br J Pharmacol* (1996) 117:170.

26 Apfelbaum M, Vague P, Ziegler O, Hanotin C, Thomas F, Leutenegger E, Long-term maintenance of weight loss after a very-low-calorie diet: a randomized blinded trial of the efficacy and tolerability of sibutramine, *Am J Med* (1999) 106:179–84.

27 Bray GA, Blackburn GL, Ferguson JM et al, Sibutramine produces dose-related weight loss, *Obes Res* (1999) 7:189–98.

28 James WPT, Astrup A, Finer N et al, for the STORM Study Group. Effect of sibutramine on weight maintenance after weight loss: a randomised trial. *Lancet* (2000) 356:2119–25.

29 Mcmahon FG, Fujioka K, Singh BN et al, Efficacy and safety of sibutramine in obese white and African American patients with hypertension – a 1-year, double-blind, placebo-controlled, multicenter trial, *Arch Intern Med* (2000) 160:2185–91.

30 Finer N, Bloom SR, Frost GS, Banks LM, Griffiths J, Sibutramine is effective for weight loss and diabetic control in obesity with type 2 diabetes: a randomised, double-blind, placebo-controlled study, *Diabet Obes Metab* (2000) 2:105–12.

31 Rissanen A, Finer N, Fujioka K, Sibutramine-induced weight loss improves lipid profile in obese type 2 diabetics: results of 3 placebo-controlled, randomized trials, *Diabetes* (2000) 49:1123.

32 Wadden TA, Berkowitz RI, Womble LG, Sarwer DB, Arnold ME, Steinberg CM, Effects of sibutramine plus orlistat in obese women following 1 year of treatment by sibutramine alone: a placebo-controlled trial, *Obes Res* (2000) 8:431–7.

33 Wilding JPH, The future of obesity treatment. In: Jolles P, ed, *New Approaches to Drug Development* (Berkhauser: Basel, 2000) 141–52.

34 Heymsfield SB, Greenberg AS, Fujioka K et al, Recombinant leptin for weight loss in obese and lean adults – a randomized, controlled, dose-escalation trial, *JAMA* (1999) 282:1568–75.

35 Williams G, Harrold JA, Cutler DJ, The hypothalamus and the regulation of energy homeostasis: lifting the lid on a black box, *Proc Nutr Soc* (2000) 59:385–96.

36 Arch JRS, Wilson S, Prospects for beta(3)-adrenoceptor agonists in the treatment of obesity and diabetes, *Int J Obes* (1996) 20:191–9.

Surgery

John G Kral

11

Introduction

There is an urgent need to address the accelerating prevalence of obesity. In the year 2000 no strategy whatsoever for primary prevention of the disease has been developed. Increasing numbers of people are entering higher obesity risk strata, with increasing incidence and severity of co-morbidity. In individuals with established obesity, co-morbidity may reverse and progression be prevented by weight loss if achieved in time and maintained indefinitely. These premises underlie acceptance of life-long drug treatment for obesity under the following conditions:

(1) The patient must respond to the treatment. 'Respond' is defined as losing and maintaining a loss of 5 or 10% of body weight over 12 weeks with maintained loss for 1 year. (Until now, only 30% of subjects are responders, regardless of type of medication.)

(2) A drug must not cause complications, side effects or adverse events that are more serious than the disease being treated – an accepted principle of risk–benefit assessment. (Long-term data on currently prescribed medications are lacking, where 'long-term' is defined

operationally as $\geq$5 years, a time span to which most people are able to relate in their daily lives.)

Surgical treatment of well-prepared, appropriate candidates, performed by competent surgeons in a proper setting, passed the risk–benefit test more than 10 years ago, with the percentage of responders well in excess of 90% using the above criteria. Furthermore, on a price per kg of weight lost basis, surgical treatment costs less than any other existing treatment after an economic break-even point of 4.5 years.[1]

Surgical treatment is underused chiefly because of the reluctance to recommend surgery to obese patients. This stems from the instinctive fear of surgery, largely based on lack of familiarity with the surgical methods, in particular their safety and efficacy. It is as natural to fear surgery as it is to deny long-term risks of serious disease or dangerous behavior such as smoking, alcoholism or weight gain. With surgery the risks are immediate and predictable, indeed scheduled. The risk of surgery is much more difficult for people to accept than any cumulative or long-term risks associated with pleasurable activity (such as overconsumption of palatable food), regardless of their understanding of the severity or probability of adverse effects. This is the crux of physicians' educational mission in many areas and is especially pertinent with regard to obesity. Once the danger of obesity

is understood, it should be easier to overcome the fear of undergoing surgery.

It is my goal in the following text to overcome some of the reluctance to recommend antiobesity surgery. On the other hand, much needs to be improved in this type of treatment before it is ready for dissemination among all-too-eager surgeon-technicians lacking the education, experience or commitment required to optimize outcomes of antiobesity surgery.

Indications for surgery

In considering the indications for surgery, it is important to keep in mind that eligibility or appropriateness as a candidate is an entirely different issue, independent of medical need. The most commonly accepted indication for surgery is based on a simple weight criterion: body mass index $\geq$40 kg/m^2. This criterion has been adopted on pragmatic grounds: at this level of weight (100 kg at 158 cm) complications are either already present or extremely likely to appear, and all nonsurgical treatment has been demonstrated to be futile. Also commonly accepted is the weight criterion of BMI $\geq$35 in the presence of serious co-morbidity demonstrated to be responsive to weight loss.

These indications originate from the period up to the mid-1980s. Subsequently significant advances in the surgical management of severe obesity have occurred as increasing evidence has demonstrated the efficacy and safety of surgical treatment, the health risks of the metabolic syndrome of obesity ('Syndrome X'), related more to distribution of fat than to body weight, and the continued failure of other treatment modalities. Under these circumstances it is not unreasonable to widen the indications for surgery with respect to simple weight criteria, especially in the presence of severe co-morbidity in the face of failed maintenance of weight control. An example might be a 40-year-old man with a syndrome of sleep apnea, hypertension and mood disorder with a BMI of 'only' 33 kg/m^2.

than a total volume of 15 ml of food, *including liquid*, at any one time will inexorably lead to vomiting. It is imperative for the patient to comprehend and learn this fact before undergoing this type of surgery. The most difficult aspect of this information for the patient is understanding that the amount of liquid must be included in the volume when any solid food is ingested. Other 'rules of eating' are listed in Table 11.1. The mechanism of action of obstructive operations is distension of the proximal gastric 'pouch' and possibly the distal esophagus, depending on the competency of the lower esophageal sphincter (LES).

Types of gastrointestinal operations

Antiobesity surgery is behavioral surgery. Despite numerous variations only two principles are employed in antiobesity surgery, though various mechanisms come into play. The procedures are either obstructive or diversionary or combinations of the two.

The most commonly performed operations worldwide are gastric restrictive obstructive procedures, termed gastroplasty or gastric banding. Placement of the constriction is so proximal in the stomach, that the capacity of the reservoir is less than 20 ml of solid food, often only 15 ml. The inner diameter of the constriction is usually less than 1 cm. This means that ingestion of more

Table 11.1
'Rules of eating' after gastric restrictive surgery.

- *Eat slowly in a quiet setting – no stress/distraction*
- *Advance diet from liquids to purées to solids*
- *Predetermine small portions*
- *Chew properly before swallowing*
- *Stop eating immediately when your pouch is full*
- *Never drink with food*
- *Wait at least 1 hour before drinking after food*

If you vomit or regurgitate:
- *Identify the reason(s)*
- *Wait 4 hours before drinking*
- *Advance diet, only if tolerated*
- *If not tolerated: contact your surgeon*

The development of inflatable circumgastric bands facilitates adjustment of stoma size via a subcutaneously implanted injectable fluid receptacle of the type used for chemotherapy or home parenteral nutrition (for example Infusaport® or Port-a-cath®). These operations can fairly easily be performed laparoscopically, significantly improving the perioperative safety of operating on severely obese patients.

Two types of diversionary operations are currently in use. The most commonly performed variant is *gastric bypass*, which is achieved by cross-stapling 15–20 ml of the most proximal stomach and connecting a limb of small intestine (jejunum) into which food and liquid can empty without first being digested by gastric or biliopancreatic secretions. Variations in pouch volume and intestinal limb length achieve different amounts of weight loss. During the first postoperative year, gastric bypass causes restriction similar to that of the purely restrictive operations, which is one of the mechanisms of weight loss. The bypass, on the other hand, interferes with digestion, exposing small bowel to undigested food which elicits sensations of fullness. This 'satiety' or nimiety (an unpleasant feeling of fullness) adds a more durable appetite regulatory mechanism to the more transitory effect of pouch distension. The maldigestion contributes to maintenance of weight loss after the first year, but affects iron, calcium and vitamin B_{12} absorption.

It is imperative that, prior to having gastric bypass, patients comprehend and learn that they will be required to take vitamin and mineral supplements for the rest of their lives after the operation and have blood tests at least annually to monitor for deficiencies.

The less commonly performed diversionary operation, called *biliopancreatic bypass (BPD)*, is similar to gastric bypass but involves removal of part of the stomach and diversion of the biliopancreatic secretions to the last portion of the small bowel (terminal ileum). Its mechanisms of action are similar to those of gastric bypass, though it causes greater maldigestion and more malabsorption. A recent modification of this operation, switching the intestinal loops, BPD/duodenal switch, has been shown to cause less malabsorption and fewer complications.[2] Nevertheless, because of the maldigestive and malabsorptive properties of these operations candidates must be able financially and logistically to submit to rigorous, knowledgeable postoperative follow-up for monitoring of their nutritional state.

Laparoscopic approaches have revolutionized all forms of surgery. Their benefits over open procedures are particularly striking in obese patients. The simpler, restrictive operations are not technically demanding and have thus been exploited to a remarkable degree in Europe and Australia, where laparoscopically placed bands are approved for general use. Laparoscopic restrictive operations are extremely safe once the surgeon has overcome the 'learning curve'. However, their efficacy is no better than that of the same operations performed openly. The important issues of patient education and preparation, and selection of appropriate candidates, are just as relevant regardless of technique.

Because of the relative ease and safety of laparoscopic restrictive surgery, including reversibility because of the nonreactive nature of the implanted bands, I have advocated a *staged* or step-care strategy for antiobesity surgery.[3] Figure 11.1 provides a classification of the severity of different operations based on type and approach, ie open or laparoscopic. Using a staged strategy, one increases the severity of the operation with documented increased severity of the eating disorder manifested in failure of the prior operation (Figure 11.2).

The magnitude of weight loss, which correlates with co-morbidity reduction and duration of maintenance, is a function of the

Immediate		Low	Long-term
Jaw wiring			Restrictive
		S	VBG
Lap	band	E	
	VBG	V	band
		E	
Open	band	R	
	VBG	I	Diversionary
		T	RYGB
Lap	RYGB	Y	
Open	RYGB		BPD/switch
Open	BPD/switch		
			Combinations
Lap	BPD/switch		RYGB + band
		High	

Figure 11.1
Immediate and long-term severity of different antiobesity operations. Lap = laparoscopic, VBG = vertical banded gastroplasty, RYGB = Roux-en-Y gastric bypass, BPD/switch = biliopancreatic bypass with duodenal switch.

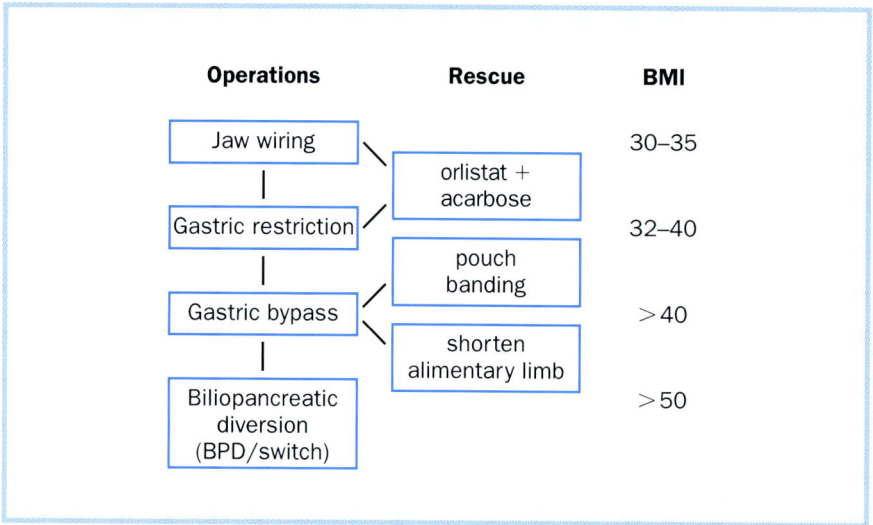

Figure 11.2
Staged or step-care strategy for antiobesity surgery. Lines between boxes denote failure of modality leading to alternative strategy (rescue). The BMI categories are arbitrary (not evidence-based): any given operation might be considered for a lower category.

'severity' or medical penalties of an operation. The majority of patients wish to lose all of their excess body weight (defined as weight in excess of actuarial standards of weight for height), regardless of the fact that lesser degrees of weight loss will ameliorate or even cure co-morbidity, improve quality of life and increase longevity. An important aspect of the preoperative educational process is to define for the patient realistic goals with respect to improvement in health and quality of life associated with the degree of weight loss achieved by various treatment options,

including different types of operations. This should be obligatory for teams providing antiobesity surgery, but unfortunately is rarely practiced because surgeons are often committed to one type of operation because they are convinced of the superiority of their routine operation or because of their limited repertoire.

Eligibility

In most settings, self-referral for surgical treatment of obesity is more frequent than professional medical referral. In part this may be due to the resistance on the part of internists alluded to earlier, and in part to ignorance about the current success of such treatment. Patients usually seek out surgical options after having repeatedly failed other methods. Their reasons for wanting surgery are related to self-perceived quality of life – more often related to psychosocial adjustment (including cosmesis) than to health. Professional referral, on the other hand, is predominantly for treatment of manifest co-morbidity (most often diabetes) and more rarely for prevention.

Candidates for surgery must fully understand the medical need for weight loss. Their understanding can be demonstrated by their ability to explain the necessity of losing weight and having a history of prior attempts to reduce. Candidates should not have psychopathology that might interfere with follow-up. This does not require psychiatric consultation because psychiatrists have not proven to have methods for predicting compliance. Lastly, it is important that candidates have sufficient resources intellectually, financially and logistically to adhere to follow-up regimens which may mean paying for blood tests and supplements, taking time off from work and traveling to a knowledgeable clinician.

The main points of eligibility are listed in Table 11.2. The 'rules of eating' (and vomiting) pertain to all gastric operations for

Table 11.2
Eligible candidates for antiobesity surgery.

- *Understand the medical need for weight loss*
- *Comprehend mechanisms of operations*
- *Understand risks and benefits of surgery*
- *Know the 'rules of eating'*
- *Have realistic expectations of long-term outcome*
- *Lack psychopathology interfering with follow-up*
- *Demonstrate reliable appointment keeping*
- *Have adequate resources for follow-up*

obesity. As emphasized earlier, the mechanism of purely restrictive procedures relates to volitional control of the ingested total volume of solid plus liquid food (≤ 15 ml). Teaching this fact often requires multiple preoperative sessions, with reinforcement postoperatively. Bypass operations require understanding of the need for life-long supplementation of vitamins and minerals combined with at least annual blood testing.

Preoperative evaluation ('medical clearance') is suggested to include the parameters listed in Table 11.3 as a minimum, in addition to the routine tests prior to any major surgery. Naturally, other tests and studies might be indicated in individual cases or in specific research protocols. Notably absent from this list are thyroid function tests, corticosteroids and pulmonary function tests, all of which have been demonstrated to be cost-ineffective performed routinely in obese patients. I have reviewed the perioperative management of obese patients, not specifically related to antiobesity surgery, in some detail in a generally available textbook,[4] to which the interested reader is referred.

Patient selection

The overall objectives of patient selection are to maximize perioperative safety and to optimize long-term outcome. The preoperative evaluation listed in Table 11.3 focuses on factors contributing to the immediate risks of operation and anesthesia rather than long-term outcome including weight loss, co-morbidity reduction, side effects and complications. It is interesting to note in this context that psychopathology is predictive of postoperative medical complications.

In an attempt to stratify risk, I suggested an 'obesity severity index' (OSI) in 1996 built on factors of physiological importance for the perioperative outcome (Table 11.4).[5] Such an index would also permit prospective evaluation of risk reduction and comparisons between different patient populations. I have now constructed a similar scale based on psychosocial factors, the obesity severity index II (Table 11.5), with the goal of predicting

Table 11.3
Preoperative evaluation for 'medical clearance' prior to antiobesity surgery.

> **Routine**
> **Blood chemistry**
> glucose
> lipids
>   triglycerides
>   cholesterol
>   HDL
> liver function
>
> **Chest X-ray**
>
> **Electrocardiogram**
>
> **As needed**
> Gastroscopy (hiatus hernia)
> Sleep study (apnea)
> Dental status
> Ear, nose, throat (obstruction)
> Psychiatric consultation

long-term co-morbidity reduction related to sustained weight loss. Just as is the case with OSI I, the items are constructed from data from published studies of predictors of 'success' in nonsurgical as well as surgical weight-loss programs. A compilation of positive and negative outcome predictors is presented in Table 11.6.

There is controversy over the importance of *binge-eating disorder* (BED) for the outcome of the different types of surgery. Some centers have suggested that it is a contraindication for antiobesity surgery, while others have demonstrated improvement or even 'cure' of BED postoperatively. The

Table 11.4
Obesity severity index I. Adding the total number of points produces a measure of severity.

Obesity severity index I: physiological maximum = 20 points			
Male sex	1	Neck:thigh > 0.70	2
Age > 40 years	1	Cardiomegaly	2
Smoker	2	Uncontrolled blood pressure	2
Sleep apnea history	1	Hemoglobin > 15 g/l	1
Thromboembolism	1	$pCO_{2 >}$ 45 mm Hg	1
Diabetes	1	Hyperinsulinemia	2
BMI 35–40 = 2; BMI > 40 = 3			

'Thromboembolism' refers to any history of the disease.
'Neck:thigh' represents the circumference ratio.

Table 11.5
Obesity severity index II. Totaling points accrued under each subheading produces a predictor of long-term weight loss failure.

Obesity severity index ii: psychosocial maximum = 20 points			
Socioeconomic	**2.0**	**Race/ethnicity/culture**	**1.0**
Education < high school grad	0.5	Black	1.0
Public insurance	0.5	Hispanic	1.0
Unmarried	0.5		
Unemployed	0.5		
		Significant co-dependent	**2.0**
Psychiatric	**7.0**		
Hospital admission	2.0	**Beliefs**	**1.5**
Manifest psychopathology	2.0	Unreasonable expectations	1.0
Abnormality on testing	1.0	Denial of disease	0.5
Childhood abuse	2.0		
		Preoperative behaviors	**2.5**
Addiction	**2.0**	Poor appointment-keeping	0.5
Alcohol	0.5	Not quit smoking	0.5
Drugs	1.5	Prior antiobesity surgery	1.5
BMI 40–50 = 1.0; BMI > 50 = 2.0			

Table 11.6
Factors influencing postoperative complication rates and outcome in severely obese subjects.

Positive	Negative
• Age < 40 years	• Prior psychiatric admission
• Employment	• MMPI psychopathology
• Married	• Prior bariatric surgery
• Social support	• Public assistance
• Appointment keeping	• Negative life events
• Realistic expectations	• Alcohol, drug use
• Diet compliance	• Snacking
• Female sex	• Black ethnicity
• Preoperative weight loss	• Co-dependent
• Education	• Secondary gain

prevalence of BED is high among severely obese patients, but large differences between populations are being reported: between 40 and 90%. I found a prevalence of 60% while participating in the original development of the scale by Spitzer et al.[6] Interestingly, when I tested the questionnaire on patients who had already had operations, all of them retrospectively qualified as having had the binge eating disorder preoperatively.

It seems intuitively logical to expect a more severe eating disorder the heavier the patient, just as co-morbidities demonstrate a dose(weight)–response relationship. Figure 11.3 shows percentile scores on the binge eating questionnaire, loosely interpreted as a measure of severity of binge eating, plotted against BMI in 16 patients (13 female, 3 male) being evaluated for antiobesity surgery. Their mean BMI was 47 ± 1.6 (SEM) with a range of 35–58. It will take a large series of patients observed for 5 or more years to determine whether these findings have predictive value.

Outcome

Weight loss after 5 years amounts to 20–25% of preoperative body weight after gastric restrictive operations, 33–38% after gastric bypass and around 40% after BPD. Weight nadir is achieved after a mean of 12 months after restrictive operations and 20–24 months after diversionary procedures. There is a gradual increase with little fluctuation over the long term after gastric restriction, while the slope of weight gain after bypass is more gradual, exhibiting some mild fluctuation beyond 3–5 years.

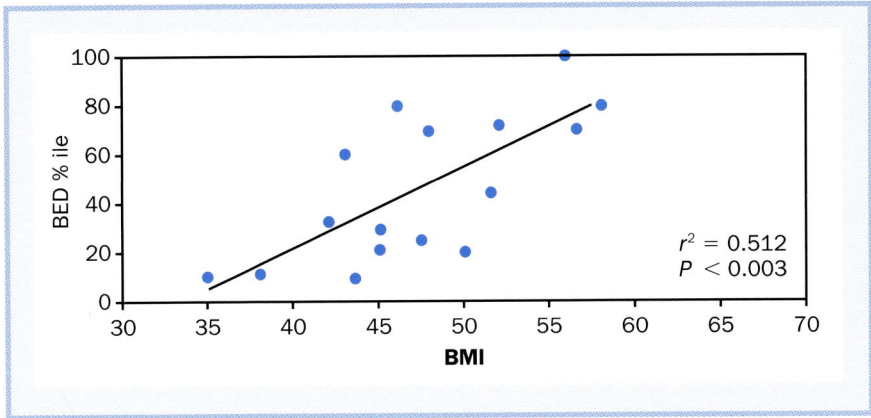

Figure 11.3
Relationship between percentile score on the binge eating questionnaire (BED %) and body mass index (BMI) in 16 (13 female, 3 male) severely obese surgical candidates.

Comorbidity reduction occurs early after all types of operations, even before there has been substantial weight loss. Most dramatic is the decline in insulin requirements and oral hypoglycemic agents in diabetics, which is virtually instantaneous after any antiobesity operation and is seen in more than 95% of patients.[7] The 5% of patients with recurrence of diabetes were older at the time of their operation and had the disease for a longer period of time than those without recurrence.

Hypertension has a 60% initial response rate, though it appears that these data erode over time. The reasons are not known, but it might be speculated that losing weight in itself has an antihypertensive effect independent of the etiology of the hypertension. When weight stabilizes this effect disappears, unveiling the intrinsic hypertension. It is likely that there are subgroups of obese hypertensive patients with varying sensitivity to obesity-related factors and to weight loss.

Numerous other co-morbid conditions have been demonstrated to be cured or ameliorated after antiobesity surgery.[3] Several malignancies are related to obesity through unknown mechanisms. It has been suggested that weight loss might have a preventive effect, but there is no evidence as yet to support this suggestion.

All surgery causes *complications*, especially in the obese, and gastrointestinal surgery is commonly associated with numerous side effects. Adhering to eligibility criteria and careful selection of surgical candidates, as implied earlier, can significantly reduce surgical morbidity and mortality. Mortality rates in centers specializing in antiobesity surgery are below 0.5%. A registry of surgeons in the USA is reporting mortality of around 0.2%.

Vomiting is a function of preoperative education, since it is totally modifiable by appropriate changes in eating behavior such as obeying the 'rules of eating'. The majority of patients who vomit after gastric restrictive operations do so for behavioral reasons and will respond to proper education. However, the purely restrictive operations with bands can develop obstructing stenosis as a complication of vomiting, nonsteroidal anti-inflammatory drug use or aggressive overeating. Vomiting must never be accepted as an expected outcome of this surgery, neither by the patient nor the physician. 'Starvation injury' can lead to fatalities.[8]

Of quantitatively greater concern after gastric restrictive operations is gastroesophageal reflux disease (GERD), because it can be insidious and over the very long term lead to serious complications. It is true that the disease is prevalent in severe obesity even before any operation, but it may become clinically manifest and progress after restrictive operations if the gastric pouch includes too much acid secretory mucosa. Between 5 and 10% of patients may ultimately require conversion of purely restrictive operations to gastric bypass, which effectively cures the esophagitis.

Gastric bypass can cause *deficiencies* in vitamin B_{12} and calcium unless supplementation is implemented immediately postoperatively and maintained for life. Obviously these deficiencies are totally preventable and their prevalence is a function of physician diligence and patient compliance. With biliopancreatic diversion/duodenal switch the risks of deficiencies are greater and include protein malnutrition. Meticulous monitoring is required. Specifics of such monitoring, focused on sequelae of gastrointestinal surgery for obesity, are reviewed by Kral.[9]

Failure to lose adequate weight and weight regain with persistence or recurrence of co-morbidity constitute indications for *reoperation.* The scheme in Figure 11.2 suggests a rescue strategy for failures of this type. Reoperations are more common after purely gastric restrictive procedures, as would be expected. Revision rates for all types of antiobesity surgery vary between 5 and 25% depending on the operation, the patient population and the attitude of the surgeon. Reoperations in general are encumbered by a higher complication rate as with all surgery. Revisional antiobesity surgery should be performed in centers with considerable experience.

Conclusions

Laparoscopic approaches have dramatically improved the safety and postoperative comfort of antiobesity surgery when performed by competent laparoscopic surgeons with experience in the field of antiobesity surgery. This should increase the use of this surgery in eligible candidates. However, the greatest effort is not related to the technical performance of one operation or another. Preoperative education and postoperative reinforcement of appropriate behavior, whether by reiterating the 'rules of eating' or monitoring the use of supplements, are the most important aspects of this surgery. If the surgeon is not personally involved in all facets of care of the individual patient, it is unlikely that an optimal outcome will be achieved.

References

1   Martin LF, Tan T-L, Horn JR et al, Comparison of the costs associated with medical and surgical treatment of obesity, *Surgery* (1995) **118**:599–607.

2   Marceau P, Hould F-S, Simard S et al, Biliopancreatic diversion with duodenal switch, *World J Surg* (1998) **22**:947–54.

3   Kral JG, Surgical treatment of obesity. In: Bray GA, Bouchard C, James WPT eds, *Handbook of Obesity* (Marcel Dekker: New York, 1998) 977–93.

4   Kral JG, Obesity. In: Lubin MF, Walker HK, Smith III RB, eds, *Medical Management of the Surgical Patient*, 3rd edn (Lippincott: Philadelphia 1995) 415–23.

5   Kral JG, Side effects, complications and problems in anti-obesity surgery: introduction of the obesity severity index. In: Angel A, Anderson K, Bouchard C et al, eds, *Progress in Obesity Research: 7* (John Libbey: London, 1996) 655–61.

6   Spitzer RL, Devlin M, Walsh BT et al, Binge eating disorder: a multisite field trial of diagnostic criteria, *Int J Eating Disord* (1992) **11**:191–203.

7   Pories WJ, Swanson MS, MacDonald KG et al, Who would have thought it? An operation proves to be the most effective therapy for adult-onset diabetes mellitus, *Ann Surg* (1995) **222**:339–52.

8   Mason EE, Starvation injury after gastric reduction for obesity, *World J Surg* (1998) **22**:1002–7.

9   Kral JG, Therapy of severe obesity. In: Haubrich W, Schaffner F, Berk JE, eds, *Bockus Gastroenterology*, 5th edn (WB Saunders: Philadelphia, 1994) 3231–9.

An integrated approach to the management of overweight and obesity

Peter G Kopelman

12

The traditional physician-centred model of care is ill suited to successful management of overweight and obesity. Obesity requires a coordination of care from multiple health care providers with a multi-disciplinary group with varied expertise working together as a team to assist patient care.

Clinical assessment

Clinical setting

The usual principles for a medical consultation are applicable to the assessment of an overweight or obese patient. The consultation room must be properly equipped with larger than average chairs, access for wheelchairs for patients with mobility problems and medical equipment of appropriate size (examination couch, blood pressure cuff, weighing scales and tape measure).

Historical background

Table 12.1 outlines the areas of medical history that should be covered at the initial assessment. The history of weight gain should be described in detail to elucidate possible aetiological factors and to assess the patient's insight and understanding of the factors causing weight gain. It is also useful to distinguish childhood onset obesity from that occurring later in life either in relation to specific physiological 'critical periods' or to illness. A number of syndromes are associated with childhood-onset obesity, but the longevity of history and the associated clinical features generally make such cases obvious (Table 12.2). Disease involving the hypothalamus can often be distinguished from 'spontaneous' or 'simple' obesity by a shorter duration of weight gain and specific symptoms related to associated endocrine disturbances. The single gene disorders involving leptin and its signalling pathways are somewhat more difficult to distinguish from simple obesity, but extreme weight gain from early childhood, a positive family history and the associated clinical features described in Table 12.2 are positive indications. The most common single gene disorder causing obesity, MC4R deficiency, is problematic as there are no pathognomonic features, but the diagnosis should be considered in cases of early-onset, familial obesity, usually with a clear dominant inheritance.[1]

The measurement of serum leptin is not recommended as a routine, but in cases of severe, early-onset obesity this should be undertaken as, although rare, congenital leptin deficiency is a potentially treatable disorder.[1]

Table 12.1
Key points to cover when taking a history from an obese patient.

- *Medical history, risk factors and established complications from obesity – enquiry about snoring and daytime somnolence*
- *Body weight history (landmarks for weight gain: puberty, employment, marriage, pregnancies, age at menopause, injuries resulting in periods of immobility, etc)*
- *History of previous treatment(s) for obesity (including successes and failures)*
- *Family history of obesity, related diseases and risk factors (ie type 2 diabetes, hypertension, premature coronary heart disease and gallstones)*
- *Diet history including usual eating pattern, alcohol intake*
- *Activity and lifestyle*
- *Relevant social history including cigarette smoking*
- *Drug history – drugs associated with weight gain, eg phenothiazines, tricyclics, anticonvulsants, lithium, anabolic and glucocorticoid steroids*
- *In women, menstrual history (irregular menses associated with polycystic ovary syndrome)*

Table 12.2
Genetic and clinical characteristics associated with monogenic causes of human obesity.

Syndrome	Locus/mode of inheritance	Obesity characteristics	Other features
Prader–Willi	15q11 Imprinted gene	Feeding difficulties at birth, followed by extreme hyperphagia and weight gain with generalized obesity from age 2–3 years. Short stature	Hypogonadism, hypotonia, small hands and feet, scoliosis, learning difficulties, behavioural problems
Bardet–Biedl	16q21, 11q13, 15q22,3p12 All recessive	Overlap with Lawrence–Moon–Bardet–Biedl (which is characterized by progressive spastic paraparesis and without polydactyly); onset of generalized obesity in first 2 years. Short stature	Retinitis pigmentosa, hypogonadism, learning difficulties, polydactyly
Cohen	8q22–23 Recessive	Truncal obesity from mid-childhood	Hypogonadism, delayed puberty with or without hypogonadism
Alstrom	2p12–13 Autosomal recessive	Normal height, truncal obesity from mid-childhood	Hypogonadism, blindness in infancy from retinal degeneration, deafness, insulin resistance, diabetes mellitus, progressive nephropathy
Edwards			Similar to Alstrom but with pigmented retinopathy
Klinefelter's	XXY	Adult onset with peripheral distribution. Tall with eunuchoid proportions	Hypogonadal, moderate learning difficulties, gynaecomastia
Albright hereditary osteodystrophy (Gs alpha mutations)	Autosomal recessive	Childhood onset	Round face, Variable hormone resistance including TSH, PTH, Short 4th metacarpal
Congenital leptin deficiency	Autosomal recessive	Childhood onset, generalized obesity, normal stature, marked hyperphagia	Hypogonadal, insulin resistance
Prohormone convertase 1	Autosomal recessive	Childhood onset – one subject described to date	Hypogonadism, Hyperproinsulinaemia, Reactive hypoglycaemia, Hypoadrenalism
Leptin receptor	Autosomal recessive	Childhood onset – three subjects described to date	Hypogonadism, Short stature, hypothyroidism
POMC	Autosomal recessive	Childhood onset – two subjects described to date	Hypoadrenalism, Red hair, Pale skin
MC4R	Autosomal dominant	~10 subjects described to date	None

Clinical examination

An outline of a scheme for the clinical examination is given in Table 12.3. Height should be measured accurately using a stadiometer and weight measured by accurate scales calibrated against known weights. Fat distribution is assessed by measurement of the waist circumference and used to refine an assessment of risk for patients with a BMI of 25 to 34.9. Waist circumference is taken as the mid-point between the lower rib margin and the iliac crest. As pointed out in Chapter 3, a waist circumference >90 cm in men and fasting plasma triglyceride levels are superior to the waist to hip ratio and BMI as screening tools for identifying abdominally obese men

with an atherogenic dyslipidaemia of insulin resistance.

An examination of the skin is important: thin, atrophic skin is a feature of corticosteroid excess; acanthosis nigricans (pigmented, 'velvety', skin creases especially in the axillae) suggests insulin resistance; severe hirsutism in women may indicate the polycystic ovary syndrome. A neck circumference of >43 cm (17 inches) indicates a likelihood of obstructive sleep apnoea (Chapter 6), while abnormal external gonadal status accompanied by intellectual impairment may suggest a rare genetic syndrome. Gastro-oesophageal reflux is a common cause of persistent cough in an obese patient.

Table 12.3
Checklist of key points for the examination and investigation of an obese patient.

Examination
- Height, weight – calculate BMI
- Blood pressure
- Neck circumference
- Any evidence for cardiac valvular disease
- Any evidence for pulmonary hypertension, cor pulmonale or congestive cardiac failure
- Signs of hyperlipidaemia
- Signs of thyroid disease
- Ophthalmic evidence for diabetes or sustained hypertension

Investigations
- Fasting blood glucose
- Fasting lipid profile
- Strip test for urine glucose and protein
- Free thyroxine and TSH

Assessment of risk

An assessment of an obese patient's absolute risk status requires an assessment of associated disease conditions (established CHD, other atherosclerotic diseases, type 2 diabetes and sleep apnoea), other obesity-associated diseases such as gynaecological abnormalities, osteoarthritis, gallstones and stress incontinence, and cardiovascular risk factors. These will include cigarette smoking, hypertension, high-risk LDL cholesterol (>4 mmol/l), low HDL cholesterol (<1 mmol/l), impaired fasting blood glucose and family history of premature CHD. Patients can be classified as being of high absolute risk if they have three of these risk factors; such patients usually require specific management of risk factors (Chapters 2 to 6).

Cigarette smoking

For the obese patient who smokes, smoking cessation is a major goal for risk management. A major obstacle to smoking cessation is the attendant weight gain. The weight gained with smoking cessation is less likely to produce negative health consequences compared to continued smoking. For this reason, smoking cessation should be strongly advocated combined with prevention of weight gain.

Assessment of motivation to lose weight

Not all patients are prepared for weight reduction despite a referral to a medical practitioner. As a consequence, it is often useful to apply the stages of change model to assess 'readiness of change' to confirm that a patient understands the need for weight loss and is prepared to follow medical advice to achieve and maintain an agreed weight goal (Chapters 7 and 8).

Integrated management

The recommendation to treat overweight and obesity is based on evidence that relates obesity to increased mortality and the results from randomized controlled trials (RCT) that demonstrate weight loss reduces risk factors for other diseases. A number of professional, governmental and other bodies have drawn up guidelines for obesity management. These strategies for providing care to the obese patient provide useful and evidence-based guidance for clinical management. An important feature of an integrated management programme is the coordination of care ensuring that a comprehensive, unified treatment plan is provided to the patient. The physician's role is to evaluate, manage and monitor, utilize adjuvant strategies when indicated (pharmacotherapy, surgery), set weight loss goals and expectations, provide support for other team members and coordinate interdisciplinary care (Figure 12.1).

illustrated by previous chapters, management frequently requires an individually-tailored approach.

Aims for a weight loss programme

Any treatment programme for overweight and obese patients should place equal importance on the problem of weight reduction and the maintenance of the lowered weight. Obesity may not respond to conventional methods of treatment such as a low-calorie diet: as

Goals of weight loss

The success or failure of a treatment programme may be judged by an arbitrarily chosen target weight or percentage weight loss. After an initial period of relatively rapid weight reduction, an average continuing loss of anything up to 1 kg per week should be

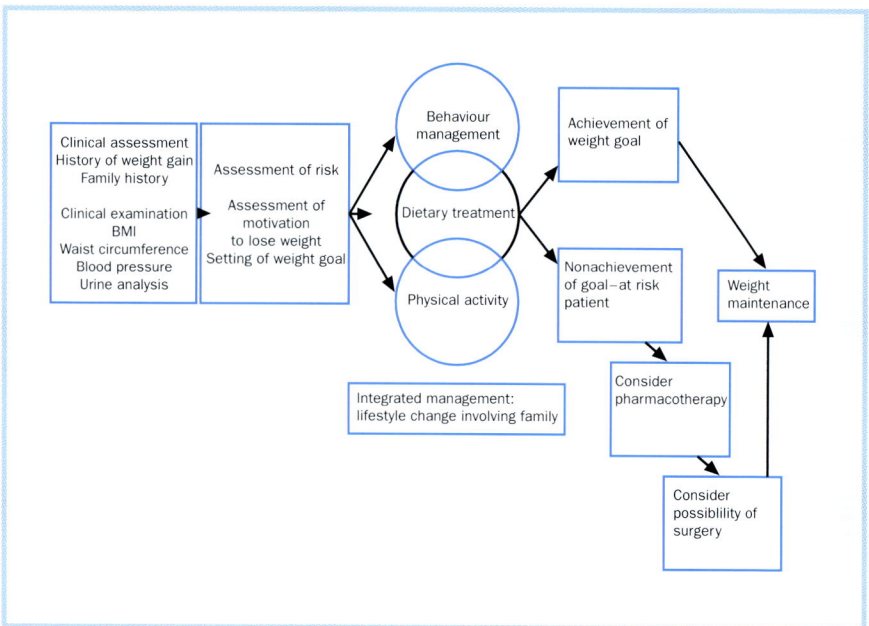

Figure 12.1
A scheme for the integrated management of overweight and obesity

considered as acceptable. Assessment of success must take account of the age of the patient, the initial degree of obesity, the presence of indicators of associated risk or complications and previous attempts at weight control. Weight loss goals for overweight and obese patients and weight goals should be tailored to the individual. A weight loss of 5% of the initial body weight will result in some improvement, while a loss of 10% is of major benefit, with clinically useful changes such as a lowered blood pressure, reduction in plasma total cholesterol and triglycerides, an increase in HDL cholesterol and a significant improvement in diabetic control (Table 12.4). The primary goal of treatment is a 10% reduction from the initial weight; successful weight loss should be regarded as a loss of more than 5%, with the consequent amelioration of risk factors; a very successful weight loss is greater than 20% in obese patients. Weight loss should be approached incrementally, with new weight loss goals negotiated with the patient if the original target is achieved. Goals for older patients (>65 years) will be different from those who are young – data suggest that a population becomes heavier with age, whereas the risk from obesity does not increase proportionately. In some patients, particularly older patients, prevention of further weight gain may be more appropriate than actual weight loss.

Dietary treatment of obesity

Chapter 7 confirms that control of diet is the cornerstone for the management of

Table 12.4
Potential health benefits that may accrue from the loss of 10 kg from the initial body weight in those patients with co-morbidities. (Adapted from Jung, British Medical Bulletin 1997,[4] with acknowledgement.)

Mortality	*20–25% fall in total mortality*
	30–40% fall in diabetes-related deaths
	40–50% fall in obesity-related cancer deaths
Blood pressure	*Fall of approx 10 mm Hg in both systolic and diastolic values*
Diabetes	*Reduces risk of developing diabetes by >50%*
	Fall of 30–50% in fasting glucose levels
	Fall of 15% in HbA1c
Lipids	*Fall of 10% in total cholesterol*
	Fall of 15% in LDL cholesterol
	Fall of 30% in triglycerides
	Increase of 8% in HDL cholesterol

overweight and obese patients. Long-term changes in food choices, eating behaviour and lifestyle are needed, rather than a temporary restriction of specific foods. The treatment should be nutritionally sound and aim to promote a healthier diet, while moderating energy intake and increasing physical activity. Such a treatment may require a period of supervision for at least 6 months. A review of 48 RCTs shows strong and consistent evidence that an average weight loss of 8% of the initial body weight can be obtained over 3 to 12 months with a low-calorie diet (LCD) and that this weight loss effects a decrease in abdominal fat.[2]

A clinician's responsibility (Chapter 7) is to judge, through assessment and discussion with their patients, which dietary strategies are relevant and to provide information and guidance in an appropriately staged manner. It is vital to translate nutritional messages into specific food changes that are practical and relevant for patients to implement over the longer term. Chapter 7 details a practical approach to estimating an individual patient's daily kilocalorie requirements. For overweight patients with a BMI in the range of 27 to 35, a decrease of 300 to 500 kcal/day will result in weight losses of about 0.25–0.5 kg per week. For more severely obese patients, with a BMI >35, deficits of 500–1000 kcal/day will lead to weight losses of 0.5–1 kg per week. After 6 months the rate of weight loss usually declines and the weight may plateau because of less

energy expenditure at the lower weight. A further adjustment of calorie intake will be indicated at this stage. Chapter 7 additionally confirms the benefits of a food diary with self-monitoring of eating and drinking. The many dietary changes necessary for successful weight loss and maintenance underline the importance of integrating behavioural change within a weight management programme.

Very-low-calorie diets (VLCDs)

The use of VLCDs should only be considered after the failure of determined attempts to lose weight with conventional restriction of normal diets. It must be recognized that these diets do not beneficially alter eating habits or weight loss for the longer term. VLCDs may occasionally be useful in the hospital setting for rapid weight loss prior to a surgical procedure. RCT evidence confirms that over the longer term (>1 year), weight loss following VLCD is no different to that of LCD.

Behaviour management

Chapter 8 succinctly describes how behaviour interventions are important for facilitating changes in an individual's lifestyle. Behaviour weight control programmes encourage patients to become more aware of their eating and physical activity, focusing on changing the lifestyle and environmental factors that are controlling their behaviour. All dietary regimens should ideally be linked to behaviour therapy: such therapy may be incorporated into self-help groups. The key difference between behavioural methods and other forms of treatment for obesity is that they lay particular emphasis on personal responsibility for initiating and maintaining treatment rather than relying on external forces. The important elements of a behavioural programme include self-monitoring, stimulus control, goal setting, problem setting, cognitive restructuring and self-rewards. Social and family support is also critical to success, not only for weight loss but also for its maintenance. Obesity requires continuous care, akin to other chronic diseases, if weight management programmes are to succeed for the longer term.

Evidence from RCTs confirms behavioural strategies reinforce changes in diet and physical activity in obese adults to produce weight losses in the range of 10% over 4 months to 1 year.[2] Longer-term follow-up shows a return to baseline weight in the absence of continuing behavioural intervention. RCT evidence suggest that behaviour therapy, when used in combination with other weight loss approaches, provides additional benefits in assisting patients to lose weight for the short term (up to 1 year): extended treatment programmes improve long-term weight maintenance. Physical activity is the strongest behavioural predictor

of weight maintenance – any form of physical activity is better than none at all.

Exercise and physical activity

Physical activity plays a key role in terms of reduced risk of early mortality and several diseases (Chapter 9). Physical activity becomes even more important as the degree of obesity diminishes and where prevention of weight gain rather than substantial weight loss is targeted. When physical activity or exercise alone is used in the treatment of obesity, weight losses are modest and average 2 to 3 kg. This weight loss, although small, exceeds that predicted if direct energy expenditure calculations are performed. For any given weight loss, the loss of fat-free mass (FFM) is less in exercising versus nonexercising subjects: this is important because FFM is the best predictor of resting metabolic rate, which is the largest contributor to total daily energy expenditure. A review of RCTs reveals strong evidence that physical activity alone in obese adults results in modest weight loss and increased cardiovascular fitness.

Many patients harbour misconceptions about the type and amount of physical activity required and this may act as a barrier to exercise adoption (Chapter 8). The suggested exercise target for adults is an accumulation of moderate physical activity (equivalent to brisk walking) on at least 5 days each week.[2] The risks from exercise are not great providing it is introduced gradually and other complications such as osteoarthritis and ischaemic heart disease are taken into account. The results from RCTs suggest that a combination of diet and exercise generally produces greater weight losses than diet alone including a decrease in abdominal fat. More importantly, subjects in the exercise group adhere to the prescribed diet better than the no exercise group. One of the most consistent findings in studies of exercise is weight maintenance, with maintenance of lost weight being seen in randomized control trials after 2 years from the start of intervention.

Drug treatment

The criteria applied to the use of an antiobesity drug are outlined in Chapter 10 and are similar to those applied to the treatment of other relapsing disorders. It is important to avoid offering antiobesity drug therapy to patients who are seeking a 'quick fix' for their weight problem.

A large number of drugs have been advocated over the years as treatment for obesity. Some of these compounds are effective, but many are ineffective. The use of drugs in the management of obesity is bedevilled by the limitations of the available published scientific evidence. It is therefore important that doctors, who use these drugs, make themselves fully familiar with either the primary literature for any drug, or an authoritative summary document.[3]

Indications for antiobesity drug treatment

It may be appropriate to consider drug treatment if, after at least 3 months of supervised diet, exercise and behavioural management, or at a subsequent review, a patient's BMI is equal to or greater than 30 kg/m^2 and weight loss is less than 10% of the presenting weight. In certain clinical circumstances it may also be appropriate to consider antiobesity drug treatment for those patients with established co-morbities whose BMI is 28 kg/m^2 or greater, if this is permitted by the drug's licence.

The initiation of drug treatment will depend on the clinician's judgment about the risks to an individual from continuing obesity: drug treatment may be particularly appropriate for patients with co-morbid risk factors or complications from their obesity. A drug should not be considered ineffective because weight loss has stopped, providing the lowered weight is maintained. However, continuation of the drug should depend on the balance between the health benefits of maintained weight and the potential adverse effects of the drug.

Prescribing antiobesity drug treatment

A review of RCTs provides good evidence that pharmacological therapy combined with diet, lifestyle modification and physical activity results in weight loss in obese adults that is significantly greater than placebo when the drugs are used for 6 months to 2 years. The experience from the use of antiobesity drugs during 12–24 month randomized controlled trials indicates that approximately 30–40% of the actively treated patients respond, as judged by a 5–10% reduction in body weight maintained over 12 months. The weight loss occurs in the 'responder' group within 12 weeks. This indicates a suitable time period when 'responders' to drug treatment can be identified and a decision taken to continue the medication. Continual assessment of drug therapy for efficacy and safety is essential. If the drug is efficacious in helping a patient to lose and/or maintain weight loss, and there are no serious side effects, it may be continued. If not, it should be discontinued. Once a weight loss target has been achieved, there should be an opportunity for renegotiation of a new target, if indicated, and/or long-term monitoring with reinforcement. *Combination therapy of two drugs is contraindicated because of concerns about safety and lack of evidence of efficacy at the present time.*

Drugs not appropriate for the treatment of obesity

There is no published evidence to suggest that bulk-forming agents (eg methyl cellulose) have any beneficial long-term action for weight reduction. Diuretics, human chorionic gonadotrophin (HCG), amphetamine, dexamphetamine and thyroxine *are not* treatments for obesity and *should not* be used to achieve weight loss. Under no circumstance should thyroxine be prescribed for obesity in the absence of *biochemically proven* hypothyroidism. Metformin and acarbose may be useful in the management of the obese type 2 diabetic patient: they have no proven efficacy for obesity alone and are not licensed for such use.

Surgical treatment of obesity

There are two operative procedures currently used for the surgical treatment of obesity: gastric restriction and gastric bypass operations (Chapter 11). Most antiobesity surgical procedures have been successfully performed laparoscopically, which reduces the requirement for sedating pain medication and facilitates prompt postoperative mobilization.

A review of evidence from RCTs confirms that surgery for obesity is an option for carefully selected patients with clinically severe obesity (BMI $\geq$ 40 or BMI $\geq$ 35, with co-morbid conditions) when less invasive methods of weight loss have failed, and the patient is at high risk for obesity-associated morbidity and mortality. The nature of the surgical procedures necessitate long-term hospital follow-up for such patients. Additionally, the option of surgery may be considered for those patients at risk from their obesity who have successfully lost weight but have a past history of repeated weight loss followed by rapid weight regain.

Management of complications

Chapters 2 to 6 underline the importance of assessing the obesity-associated risk of a patient and integrating the management of the disease complication (or risk factor) within the weight management programme. Reduction of visceral fat is a main priority for the metabolic syndrome and associated cardiovascular risk. Chapter 2 highlights the potential reversibility of diabetes if weight loss is instigated early enough in management and the patient convinced of its benefits. In established type 2 diabetes, modest weight loss improves glycaemic control for the short term, whereas major weight loss (usually achieved through surgery) drastically reverses hyperglycaemia for the longer term. Chapters 3 and 4 underline the importance of treating the associated risk factors (dyslipidaemia, hypertension and cardiac failure) while awaiting anticipated benefits from weight reduction. Chapter 6 stresses the importance of fat deposition in the neck, upper airway, chest wall and abdomen in impairing respiratory mechanical function. There must be high awareness of the association of obstructive sleep apnoea with obesity, and a recognition that the early initiation of CPAP may result in considerable symptomatic well-being and concomitant improvement in an ability to lose weight.

Weight maintenance

Obesity results in most patients, not from an inability to lose weight but from a profound difficulty in maintaining a lowered weight. A programme to enable the individual to maintain their lowered weight must follow any successful weight loss. Published evidence suggests that a combination of sensible eating, physical activity and reinforcement of behavioural methods is most successful for the longer term. Clinical care can reinforce their importance, but the ultimate responsibility for following such advice must lie with the patient and the duration of follow-up tailored accordingly. Follow-up review should always include an assessment of any associated co-morbidities.

References

1   Barsh GS, Farooqi IS, O'Rahilly S, Genetics of body weight regulation: applications and opportunities, *Nature* (2000) **404**:644–51.

2   Clinical Guidelines, National Heart, Lung and Blood Institute web site: *http://www.nhlbi.nih.gov/nhbli/cardio/obes/profgu idelns/ob_gdlns.htm.*

3   *Clinical Management of Overweight and Obese Patients with Particular Reference to the Use of Drugs* (Royal College of Physicians: London, 1998).

4   Jung RT, Obesity as a disease, *Br Med Bull* **53**:307–21.

Index

Note: Page numbers in *italics* refer to figures or tables in the text